MEDICAL MENTORING

t do

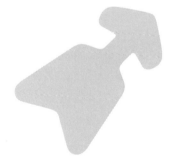

MEDICAL MENTORING

Supporting students, doctors in training and general practitioners

David Jeffrey

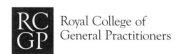

Royal College of General Practitioners

The Royal College of General Practitioners was founded in 1952 with this object:

'To encourage, foster and maintain the highest possible standards in general practice and for that purpose to take or join with others in taking steps consistent with the charitable nature of that object which may assist towards the same.'

Among its responsibilities under its Royal Charter the College is entitled to:

'Diffuse information on all matters affecting general practice and issue such publications as may assist the object of the College.'

British Library Cataloguing-in-Publication Data
A catalogue record for this book is available from the British Library

© Royal College of General Practitioners, 2014

Published by the Royal College of General Practitioners, 2014
30 Euston Square, London NW1 2FB

Disclaimer

This publication is intended for the use of medical practitioners in the UK and not for patients. The authors, editors and publisher have taken care to ensure that the information contained in this book is correct to the best of their knowledge, at the time of publication. Whilst efforts have been made to ensure the accuracy of the information presented, particularly that related to the prescription of drugs, the authors, editors and publisher cannot accept liability for information that is subsequently shown to be wrong. Readers are advised to check that the information, especially that related to drug usage, complies with information contained in the *British National Formulary*, or equivalent, or manufacturers' datasheets, and that it complies with the latest legislation and standards of practice.

Designed and typeset by Typographic Design Unit

Printed by Hobbs the Printers

Indexed by Susan Leech

ISBN: 978-0-85084-354-5

To medical students.

And when I remembered all that I hoped and feared as I picked about Rutherford's in the rain and the east wind: how I feared I should be a mere shipwreck, and yet timidly hoped not; how I feared I should never have a friend, far less a wife, and yet passionately hoped I might; how I hoped (if I did not take to drink) I should possibly write one little book I should like the incident set upon a brass plate at the corner of that dreary thoroughfare, for all students to read, poor devils, when their hearts are down.

ROBERT LOUIS STEVENSON
Letters from South Seas

___ Contents

___Preface

It is difficult to understand why some doctors who take so much care of their patients fail to extend the same level of concern to students, trainees or their peers. It is likely that all doctors struggle at some time in their careers either before or after graduation. Medical education can be perceived as competitive and stressful both in the undergraduate years and during training to become a general practitioner.

I have been fortunate to have enjoyed a twenty-year career as a general practitioner and to have had the opportunity to specialise in palliative medicine. Latterly, I worked as an Academic Mentor in the Medical School at the University of Dundee. This experience has convinced me of the central role of a mentor in providing support, encouragement and guidance to students and colleagues.

I have been lucky to have found inspirational clinical mentors during my career. It is good to reflect on the impact that these mentors have had on my own professional development. I have included a quote from them at the beginning of each chapter. Clinical teachers who take an interest in students as individuals and who are prepared to give extra time to help are never forgotten. Doctors who share their sense of vulnerability enable students to become caring doctors. I can recall students who described some of their teachers as 'terrifyingly competent' and so seemed unapproachable to a struggling student.

This book is intended for colleagues who mentor and support medical students, doctors in training or general practitioners, or who are thinking of taking up a mentoring role. Most commonly mentoring forms part of one's role as a clinician, tutor, supervisor or teacher. This guide adopts a practical approach based on a clinical model and illustrated by case studies. The case studies are fictional to preserve confidentiality but are an amalgam of true stories of struggling students and doctors in difficulty.

One of the biggest challenges in clinical care is to see the world through the patient's eyes. Students and doctors in training are not patients, they are colleagues, but part of the mentor's role is to understand their view and to give them time and space. Similarly in supporting doctors in difficulty a mentor can use his or her clinical skills to connect, communicate, listen, identify problems, and work out a plan together to help. Clinicians use these skills instinctively every day in their work with patients; they just need to adapt the same skills to support their colleagues. There are many parallels between clinical care and mentoring colleagues, and some important differences. In both situations people are facing a crisis and there is often only one opportunity to intervene to help. If concerns are to be addressed effectively the doctor needs to 'see behind the brave face'. Just as the clinician considers the 'whole' patient in reaching a diagnosis and negotiating a treatment plan, so the mentor needs to take account of both the academic and pastoral aspects of the mentee's problems. Mentoring is a developing relationship in which both mentor and mentee can gain self-awareness and develop as professionals.

At present the NHS has been described as in crisis. In the wake of the Francis Report, politicians and the media have heaped criticism on healthcare staff, in particular general practitioners.* There is little acknowledgement of the hard work and commitment of the majority of NHS staff. I hope this book will play a part in inspiring doctors to take on a mentoring role and support colleagues. Mentoring is a practical and effective way of providing this help.

Author's note

The case studies described in the book are fictional to preserve confidentiality. They are an amalgam of true stories of struggling students and doctors in difficulty.

---

* Francis R. *Report of the Mid Staffordshire NHS Foundation Trust Public Inquiry.* London: Stationery Office, 2013, www.midstaffspublicinquiry.com [accessed 25 June 2014].

___ *Foreword*

As doctors, we are our own most useful tools. Being able to connect, to empathise, to hear, to imagine, to think, to theorise, to test, to plan and to educate are essential skills, and they are skills of the self, of being human. It should go without saying that, if we don't keep ourselves sharp, we won't be much use to our patients or colleagues.

So it is ironic, perhaps even tragic, that so few of us properly care for ourselves, let alone allow our colleagues to care for us. It is an enduring mystery that doctors, who can be so caring, compassionate and skilful with their patients, can be so uncaring, cold and unskilful with ourselves. We are constantly right up there in the charts of the most depressed, most burnt-out and most addicted professions on our planet.

But we also have such an amazing job, full of interest, challenge, opportunities to connect and chances to learn. So we are also right up there in the charts of the best professions on the planet.

Sometimes, maybe most of the time, we need help to pull ourselves out of our hole and see things properly. That's where mentoring is such a wonderful thing. It enables us to turn the skills we use for our patients to the benefit of our colleagues and of ourselves. Who better to learn from than a valued colleague? Who better to turn to, to model oneself on, and to learn with, than someone who does what we do?

This wonderful book suggests that seeking mentoring should not be seen as a weakness, but rather as an essential part of professional learning and development. It shows how we can all be mentors, and how we can all benefit from being mentored. It argues persuasively that mentoring *should not be an optional extra, but rather should become an integrated and fundamental part of medical practice.*

David's work, easy to read, packed with practical case examples, and ordered in an accessible way, demystifies mentoring and shows us that it can be done pretty much by anyone, for anyone.

Ultimately, it is simply about skilful caring and that, after all, is what we do for a living!

JUSTIN AMERY

_Acknowledgements

I would like to acknowledge the help I have received from my mentors during my career. I remember these inspiring mentors for their encouragement and support in times of difficulty: John Munro, James Syme, Derek Doyle, Ted Sever, Gerry Collee, Geoff Hanks, Bill Astley, Huw Richards, 'Raj' Rajagopal, Jim Moore, Bobbie Farsides, Sean Elyan and Marie Fallon.

I am grateful to Gillian Nineham for her belief in this book and for her patience and wisdom. Thanks to the publishing team at the Royal College of General Practitioners and especially Helen Farrelly, Tony Nixon and Rodger Charlton for their advice and help. I am grateful to Justin Amery for sharing insights into general practice and for contributing a foreword to this book. I acknowledge my gratitude to Joy Hinson for permission to include an example of her innovative teaching and support. Thanks to Rob Jarvis and Alison Gillan for happy times devising practice OSCEs.

My thanks to the medical students I had the privilege of working with at Dundee Medical School, for their courage, patience and humour.

My thanks as always to Pru, my wife, for everything.

SUPPORT → 1

"I only have one rule for junior doctors: if a nurse calls you at night, you must go to the ward. There are two possibilities: either the patient is ill or the nurse is worried. Both deserve your attention."

Dr John Munro, induction chat to his new house officers

The mentor offers support to the mentee both in his or her academic and personal life. Mentoring is a part of a network of support available to students and doctors. The individual may access a number of different sources of support that meets his or her particular needs. For instance a student may be seeing a personal tutor, a mentor and a counsellor. This mix of support can vary over time as the individual matures and circumstances change.[1]

Students need to acquire skills in self-directed learning, which may require encouragement and support. There is a need to achieve a balance between autonomy and dependence. At present support tends to be provided in a reactive way following a failure; earlier, proactive support should be available to struggling students before they fail. Students want an opportunity to reflect on their academic performance and to discuss the factors that enhance or impair their progress. They wish to identify gaps in their learning and ways of meeting their learning needs. They need to reflect on the broader context of their university life and to engage in a learning community.

Examples of effective support include:

- providing easy access for face-to-face meetings with their tutor, at least twice a year

- encouraging students to access guidance and advice to achieve their full potential

- providing individual support of study skills

- providing clear information to students on available support networks, including peer support

1

- raising awareness of the student counselling and local GP services

- providing guidance on the core curriculum, optional components and assessment methods

- providing regular and prompt feedback on their academic development

- providing sample exam questions for practice purposes

- encouraging struggling students to keep in regular email contact with their tutor.

___ Transitions

Support is most often required at transition points in the doctor's career. The first transition occurs when the student must adapt to the change from school to university life. Some students cling to learning styles that worked for school exams but are not so effective for the deeper level of understanding required by medical studies.

The next transition occurs when there is a sharp division between pre-clinical and clinical years. The first exposure to patients, relatives and clinical staff on the wards can bring further stresses.

A further transition occurs when the student begins to adopt the values of a doctor, a change that usually occurs before graduation. There comes a point in the course when the student appreciates what it is to be a good doctor and absorbs the appropriate ethical and professional attitudes. This is almost an 'epiphany' and is readily recognisable to colleagues. It has something to do with an inner self-belief, humility and a commitment to putting the patient's needs first. A mentor can help facilitate this transition by acting as a role model, sharing his or her own difficulties and by treating students as colleagues.

Informal mentoring, where someone acts as a mentor without realising it, either as a role model or even sometimes taking it upon themselves to advocate for a trainee, can be a most inspiring and positive form of mentoring. The newly qualified doctor faces another transition in becoming a Foundation doctor in training for two years. He or she finds a new sense of responsibility and the sense of fulfilment that comes from using the skills learnt at university. However, pressure of work, lack of time and breaks in continuity may all lead to a sense of frustration and stress. A mentor, not involved in academic assessment, can provide vital support that supplements the role of the educational supervisor.

Specialist training involves choices of career, new responsibilities and further professional development and transitions. Mentors who have been through these experiences can guide and advise their mentees.

Specialist trainees (ST3) entering general practice may find that their hospital-based training has not equipped them fully for working in the practice setting.

General practice has been subject to enormous change over the past decade. Commissioning health care for patients, part-time working, out-of-hours services, targets and the implementation of guidelines have altered family medicine radically. General practitioners have been subject to criticism from the press and media for their performance, which only adds to stress and lowers morale. Mentoring should be an effective mechanism of providing support to general practitioners but, at present, it is often only provided once a doctor has encountered difficulties.

There are a number of transition points during a general practitioner's career. Entering practice as a qualified general practitioner is a challenging moment. Newly appointed GPs can feel out on their own without the backing of an educational supervisor or mentor. They may spend some time as a salaried partner before entering full partnership, which is yet another important transition that brings different duties and obligations.

Many GPs experience another change when they reach their forties. There may be a sense of 'What next?' They are established in the practice but face the daunting prospect of another twenty or twenty-five years of doing the same work.

The fifth decade can also be a point of transition. The GP may look forward and think, 'What can I do now to maximise benefit over the last ten years of work?' They may seek to diversify into taking on administrative or teaching roles and value a source of advice, which a mentor can provide.

Approaching retirement is difficult for many general practitioners. They may have a feeling of 'When do I go?' They may not think of a mentor as the person they could approach yet he or she might provide just the support and advice they need.

___ Undergraduate support

Many students struggle because they lack effective support.[2] The purpose of a student support scheme is to facilitate the student's development, to ensure that his or her undergraduate years are a positive experience and to help the student develop relationships that may be beneficial in the future. Student support schemes are aimed to meet the needs of all students, not just those with problems.

___ Why support medical students?

Effective support for medical students is essential, not only to create an environment that favours learning but also to avoid students leaving the course. Failing students risk disruption to their studies and may lead them to developing into doctors with problems. Investing in student support may save money as there is a significant cost if a medical student fails to qualify as a doctor. Providing support for medical students is also part of the General Medical Council (GMC) requirements of a medical school.[3]

___ An ethos of support

The philosophy of the university with regard to providing support can vary. Students are encouraged to be self-directed in their learning yet there is a risk that they may fail if left entirely to fend for themselves. Coping with uncertainty and stress is part of being a good doctor but it is still essential that all students and doctors have access to support.

Case story **Paul**

Paul, a medical student at a university with an emphasis on problem-based learning (PBL), comes to his mentor for a routine review meeting. The mentor notices he is quieter than usual and asks, 'How are things going with the course?'

Paul says he is finding his current project difficult to complete on time. The mentor is quiet and listens.

Paul goes on. 'Well it's the PBL stuff. Two guys are in the rugby team so they just leave it to us. Our supervisor has told us that our project on living with diabetes is backed up with online guidance but I don't know what level of detail she expects.'

The mentor asks Paul what he feels would help. Paul replied, 'I think it would be great to meet the supervisor, to understand what she expects us to cover. I just feel that I am working in the dark.'

The mentor asks if Paul would find it helpful for her to let the supervisor know that the group is struggling a bit and need more guidance. Paul feels relieved and is grateful for the support. The mentor asks Paul to email her next week after she has had a chance to discuss the issues with the PBL supervisor.

An inadequately supported PBL group is an example of bad educational practice. Good learning practice occurs in universities which acknowledge that they share a responsibility when a student fails. In this culture students are regarded as expected to qualify and failures as opportunities to learn and a part of progress. Support is seen to be an essential ingredient of education and all students are expected to access support, not just those who are struggling.

___ Accessing support

Students usually only seek help when things go wrong, for instance when they fail an exam. Proactive support should be available to all struggling students before they fail. It would be helpful to emphasise that such help is available to each student group at the beginning of each academic year. Indeed, accessing support should be seen as good professional behaviour; too often medical students are reluctant to seek support as they feel they will be regarded as inadequate or weak. It sometimes helps to improve access by reminding students how bad doctors are at looking after themselves, as evidenced by their high rates of alcoholism and burnout.[4,5]

Case example **innovative teaching and the importance of student support**

One innovative, light-hearted and possibly controversial approach to raising students' awareness of the importance of support is to tell them 'how to get thrown out of medical school'! This is a compelling way of illustrating unprofessional behaviour. Topics for discussion include: getting a criminal record (and hiding it from your medical school); forging a signature; alcohol and drug misuse; plagiarism; just disappearing; stopping attendance at college; not telling anyone you have a problem that interferes with your studies and then failing exams; and finally not accessing support when you need it. Discussion around these topics can be used to deepen an understanding of fitness to practise issues and help dispel myths. Students learn that the majority of referrals to a Fitness to Practise Committee are the result of either frank dishonesty or stupidity, but that most students who do get 'thrown out' of medical school are those with difficulties who do not seek help and so just fail exams. Students are encouraged to disclose problems since it is their attempt to conceal them that results in academic failure and having their studies terminated. The session is concluded by emphasising how much the medical school wants students to access support.[6]

___ Systems of undergraduate support

Mentoring is part of a package of support on offer to medical students. Universities have generic student support schemes open to all students. These include counselling, finance, health, accommodation, occupational health and disability support (see Box 1.1). It is important that a mentor has an in-depth knowledge of these generic support services and knows which ones are most appropriate for the student seeking support.

Box 1.1 **Sources of support for medical students**

- Personal tutor.
- Student counselling service.
- Student health service.
- General practitioner.
- Disability services.
- Mental health services.
- Accommodation services.
- Student finance.

- International advice service.
- Nightline.
- Samaritans.
- Academic skills centre.
- Careers service.
- Peer connections.
- Occupational health.

The generic support system in some ways mirrors the NHS in that it is constructed in a context of almost infinite needs of medical students, just as the NHS faces the escalating needs of patients. The success of any support system depends on the underlying ethos of the university towards its students.

Most universities have a support team that coordinates student support. Such a team is available to help with complex problems and will have regular review meetings to discuss the progress of struggling students. Support is commonly based on a system where each student is allocated a personal tutor or mentor.

The main elements of any effective medical ___ student support system

The following factors are required for an effective system of support for medical students:

- allowing easy access for face-to-face meetings with a tutor or mentor, at least twice a year

- encouraging students to access guidance and advice to achieve their full potential

- providing individual support of study skills

- providing clear information to students on available support, including peer support

- raising awareness of the generic student support services and local GP services

- providing guidance on the core curriculum, optional components and assessment methods

- providing regular and prompt feedback on student academic development

- providing opportunities to practise exam techniques

- encouraging struggling students to keep in regular contact with their mentor.

Case story Morag

Morag is a third-year student who has received feedback from her tutor on a case study she had written on the care of a dying patient in hospital. She comes to her mentor distressed because she only achieved a low grade.

Morag seems withdrawn and resigned, and says she always does badly in her essays but scores highly in clinical examinations. The mentor looks carefully at her case study. The ideas are good but the paragraphs do not link together in a coherent way, making the essay seem rather slapdash.

The mentor said, 'Morag, I know you are a bright student. Is there anything else worrying you?'

Morag becomes tearful. 'I have to go back home every weekend to help look after my grandfather who is unwell with heart failure and is living on his own. I am worried that he is going to die. But I had poor essay marks before he became unwell.'

The mentor listens to Morag's concerns and finds out that she has a supportive family and a boyfriend whom she can confide in. She asks Morag, 'Has anyone ever raised the possibility that you might have a form of dyslexia?'

Morag says she had been tested in school but nothing was found.

The mentor said, 'Look, I am no expert on dyslexia and clearly you do not have anything obviously wrong with your writing, but I am concerned about your ability to link ideas in a logical way. Would you like to see an expert on dyslexia who could give you a proper assessment?'

Morag is keen to get this help. The mentor spoke to the dyslexia adviser who saw Morag two weeks later and confirmed that she had a form of dyslexia. She made helpful suggestions to improve her essay writing. Morag also consented to the mentor making a note of her difficulty in her student record and gave permission for her block tutor on her attachment in care of the elderly to be made aware of her worries about her grandfather.

Morag met her mentor after a month to review her progress and was much more settled and happy in her studies. They agreed to keep in touch by email and meet if Morag wished, or at their regular end of semester meeting.

___ Challenges for student support services: an overview

These brief notes are an overview of some of the challenges facing a student support system wishing to meet the needs of medical students. Each of these areas is explored in more detail in the subsequent chapters.

Awareness of student support services

Many students are unaware of the support services that are available. Student support should not be viewed as a remedial service by the university or by students. The students need to meet their mentor at an early stage of their course. It may be helpful to have an introductory lecture on student support as an integral part of student induction. The students also need to know the key medical administrative staff who play a vital role in providing day-to-day advice on the course. The administrative staff, like everyone else involved in student support, should present a friendly face to students. The university should provide a clear directory of student support services with instructions on how to access them.

Identifying struggling students

Any support system may fail to identify students who are struggling until they fail exams. Helpful ways of addressing this problem are dealt with in Chapter 4.

Providing continuity of support

It is often difficult to maintain contact with students who are away from the university on electives or attachment to rural units. Such times may be stressful for the student, who may feel lonely away from their friends and without informal support.

8

The pressure of the curriculum may make it difficult to find a mutually convenient time for support meetings with the mentor. Some students may be reluctant to meet a mentor who is also involved in their assessment. This is discussed in more detail in Chapter 3.

Establishing boundaries

It is important that the student and mentor agree the boundaries of their availability and preferred method of contact. There is a need to emphasise that mentoring is a relationship that requires engagement by both parties. If a meeting is anticipated to be particularly difficult it may on occasion be helpful, with the student's consent, to have two mentors present.

Individual and group meetings

Individual face-to-face meetings are the core of mentoring. Students will rarely disclose real difficulties in a group. There may be coaching activities that can be dealt with in groups but never personal issues.

Space

If students are to feel less inhibited in disclosing personal difficulties there has to be a quiet, safe space for them to do so. They need privacy and time free from interruption.

Retention and motivation of students

On occasions student may have to withdraw temporarily from the course, maybe for health reasons or family crises. They should be advised to keep in contact by email with their mentor and feel part of the learning community. Some medical schools supply students with a student pack with details on how to approach their year out and how to prepare for their return. The student is expected to see their GP or specialist if they have withdrawn on health grounds.

Mental health

Providing appropriate support to students with mental health problems is essential. The subject is explored in full in Chapter 9. General practitioners and the university's occupational health department play a central role in helping students with health problems.

Some medical schools give students with health problems a laminated card that they can show to supervisors. This flags up that the student is seeing the support services and suitable allowances should be made. The supervisor can contact the lead in student support. This saves the student explaining health issues repeatedly to supervisors and the card can act as a 'safety net'.[7]

Breaches of professional behaviour by students

Students learn from the outset of their studies the standards and values expected of them as a professional.[3] Serious breaches of professional behaviour such as criminal behaviour are referred to a Fitness to Practise Committee. The mentor may have a role in advising the student and acting as his or her advocate in such hearings, especially if termination of the student's studies is being considered.

Recruiting, supporting and training mentors

Clinicians are busy people and may be unwilling to sacrifice time for a mentoring role. New mentors require training and they should have someone with whom they can discuss the complexities of their role. It is helpful if there is a forum where mentors can meet to share concerns.

Students and mentors need clear guidelines as to what they can expect from each other; sometimes this is formalised as a learning contract.

Coaching and feedback

Students are always asking for more feedback on their work and progress. Mentors should be skilled in providing feedback that is positive and constructive. The student and mentor can then devise a number of specific, achievable goals to work towards before their next meeting. Peer mentoring can also be an effective way of coaching and giving feedback.

Special groups of students

Certain student groups share difficulties: international students face language and cultural issues, widening-access students may find it hard to integrate into the course and graduate students may have difficulty juggling a work–life balance.

Some medical schools have a 'buddying system' where some students in the years above act as 'parents' for new students as they settle in. Such 'buddies' may act as peer mentors.

Confidentiality

Maintaining confidentiality is always a challenge for both the mentor and the student, who should understand its limits. Generally if there is a serious mental health problem that threatens patient care or the life of the student, or if there is a serious breach of professional behaviour that might involve fitness to practise issues, then the mentor has an obligation to share the information with the academic authorities.

Support for trainees

Support for doctors in training must be provided to prevent drop-out, to make training enjoyable and to nurture good professional development.

Case story James

James has recently been appointed as a Foundation Year 1 doctor in a new area. He meets his consultant and educational supervisor, who emphasise the importance of attending the training seminars on the medical unit. James is often late for ward rounds and he is bossy with the nurses on the ward. A patient has now complained to the consultant that James was rude to her. The consultant sees James and asks him if he sees any problem with his performance.

James replies, 'No, I seem to get along fine. The patient who complained was a poor historian and was taking so much time. I just asked her to stop waffling and to answer my questions to the point. If there is a problem on the unit it is with some of the nurses who think they know everything.'

The consultant suggests that James has a chat with his educational supervisor who has time allocated to discuss the issues in more detail (*continued below*).

The transition from undergraduate to Foundation Doctor is challenging because there are new responsibilities and pressures from work. These challenges have increased because the trainee is often working in a strange environment with new colleagues and without the support of friends and family. This is a point at which trainees may feel unsupported, isolated and stressed. They may have to balance a busy job with their home lives, and in some cases they may be being bullied.

In some ways the response to transition is similar to that of someone sustaining a loss. Clinicians are familiar with the range of emotions and behaviours accompanying grief and loss. They need to be aware that colleagues may demonstrate a similar pattern in response to change. There may be Shock, Denial, Anger, Bargaining before Acceptance and moving on.[8] A trainee may be withdrawn and show a lack of enthusiasm or, as in the case above, deny there is a problem. Anger may be shown in any number of ways; there can be a sense of frustration following a poor performance. As trainees move between these stages they may display uncharacteristic behaviours and emotions that impact on their work and their ability to communicate with patients, families and colleagues.[9]

There are a number of sources of support for doctors in training, some of which are listed in Box 1.2.

Box 1.2 **Sources of support for trainee doctors**

- Educational supervisor.

- Mentor.

- Clinical supervisor.

- Training programme director.

- Foundation programme director.

- Health Education England or deanery in Scotland.

- General practitioner.

- British Medical Association.

- Defence organisations.

- National Clinical Assessment Service (NCAS).

- Occupational health.

- Sick Doctors Trust.

___ Role of mentors for trainees

Foundation Year doctors may be confused about the difference between a mentor and an educational supervisor. Mentoring is different from educational supervision in that a mentor should not have an assessment role. The reason for this is that once trainee doctors feel that they are being assessed they may not disclose difficulties that they fear might adversely affect their career progress. Educational supervisors may have a mentoring role but the main aim of educational supervision is to maintain standards of training.[9] A mentor can provide additional pastoral support, promote professional attitudes and help with career advice.

Case story James (continued)

James sees his educational supervisor, who senses there is much more going on in James's story than just settling into a new job. He asks James if he would like to speak to a mentor with total confidentiality and who is not involved in his assessment.

James meets another consultant, who listens to James's story and asks him about adverse life events. After some time James admits that he is struggling with the new job, has little time to relax and is not sleeping. He is also drinking alcohol most evenings to try to get to sleep. He wonders whether he has made a dreadful error in choosing to become a doctor.

The mentor asks whether he is depressed. James replied, 'Yes, I do feel low. Some days I have great difficulty getting out of bed and going to work ... I just dread the ward.'

The mentor arranges for James to see a general practitioner as he was not registered with one in the area. He advises James also to see a doctor in the occupational health department of the hospital. He praises James for seeking help and reassures him that once he felt better he would be in a position to make decisions about the future. At present the main priority is his health and he needs help with his depression. The mentor suggests keeping in contact by email and a further meeting once James has seen the GP.

___ Support for general practitioners

General practitioners have come under close scrutiny by the public, media and politicians. The drive for accountability and rising patient expectations have created pressures for GPs so it is appropriate to examine the provision of support for GPs.[10]

General practitioners in difficulty cannot provide the best standards of care. GPs, like other doctors, are subject to stress, burnout, and physical and mental illnesses.[11] Starting in general practice can be a difficult transition for the specialty trainee. Doctors are generally reluctant to admit that they are struggling because they can feel that this is a sign of failure. Mentors can help GPs affected by change in either their personal or professional life when this impacts on their patient care. Stress can be caused by a number of factors: practice reorganisations, complaints, family problems and alcohol misuse. Revalidation is one way in which doctors can demonstrate that they are fit to practise and may help to identify more doctors who require further support. General practitioners also take part in annual appraisal.

However, the Local Revalidation Teams and appraisals are concerned with making judgements about the doctor's performance at work. It is unlikely that doctors are going to discuss problems such as alcohol misuse or burnout in these arena. Mentoring could help to fill a gap and provide support in a non-threatening way, and in so doing perhaps avoid more serious problems from developing. General practitioners are much more likely to discuss their real concerns on a confidential one-to-one basis with a trusted colleague they have chosen than with a responsible officer on a revalidation team. This would be an effective way to reduce the number of doctors appearing before the GMC. Some sources of support available for GPs are listed in Box 1.3.

Box 1.3 Support available for GPs

- Colleague.

- Mentor.

- British Medical Association.

- Medical defence organisations.

- GMC.

- NCAS.

- Postgraduate Medical and Dental Education (Health Education England).

- Appraisal.

- Revalidation.

___ Mentoring systems

Healthcare organisations are responsible for developing policies and procedures to recognise concerns about a GP's performance and to act to address those concerns. Two excellent initiatives illustrate that it is possible to institute effective mentoring that is appreciated by general practitioners.

The West Midlands Deanery Professional Support Unit (PSU) is targeted at doctors in difficulty.[11] This scheme offered GPs trained mentors who provided confidential peer support. Mentees were made aware from the outset that, if issues arose that directly compromised patient safety, the mentor would have to refer the matter on to the appropriate authority, which could be the GMC. These issues are discussed in Chapter 4.

The Career Development Unit (CDU) covers the Thames Valley within Health Education Thames Valley.[12] Alongside its provision of career guidance the CDU provides coaching and mentoring for doctors who self-refer or are referred. The CDU provides guidance and workshops to help educators manage performance issues in trainees, and also collaborates with trainers to provide personal coaching or mentoring for individual trainees who need additional support to improve their performance.

___ Conclusions

This chapter has reviewed the support available to students, doctors in training and general practitioners. The next chapter focuses on mentoring, a more specific way of supporting these colleagues.

Key points

Mentoring is part of a network of support.

Mentors need to know what support is available in their organisation.

The reasons behind a poorly performing student or doctor are usually complex.

Mentoring should not involve assessment.

Confidentiality is crucial in any form of support.

Transition points can cause stress and require support.

___ References

1 McKimm J, Jollie C, Hatter M, London Deanery. *Mentoring: theory and practice.* London: Faculty Development, www.faculty.londondeanery.ac.uk/e-learning/feedback/files/Mentoring_Theory_and_Practice.pdf [accessed 25 June 2014].

2 Dick J, Dixon R, Jeffrey D, McDonald L. *Getting Started … Struggling Students.* Dundee: Centre for Medical Education, University of Dundee, 2013.

3 General Medical Council. *Tomorrow's Doctors.* London: GMC, 2009.

4 Black L F, Monrouxe L V. 'Being sick a lot, often on each other': students' alcohol-related provocation. *Medical Education* 2014; **48(3)**: 268–79.

5 Maslach C. Job burnout: new directions in research and intervention. *Current Directions in Psychological Science* 2003; **12**: 189–92.

6 Hinson J. Personal communication.

7 Raven P W, Griffen A E, Hinson J P. Supporting students with disabilities using a 'student support card' scheme. *Medical Education* 2008; **42(11)**: 1142–3.

8   Hay J. *Transactional Analysis for Trainers*. Watford: Sherwood Publishing, 1996.

9   Cooper N, Forrest K. *Essential Guide to Educational Supervision in Postgraduate Medical Education*. London: BMJ Books, Wiley-Blackwell, 2009.

10 Lake J. Doctors in difficulty and revalidation: where next for the medical profession? *Medical Education* 2009; **43(7)**: 611–12.

11 Taylor CJ, Houlston P, Wilkinson M. Mentoring for doctors in difficulty. *Education for Primary Care* 2012; **23(2)**: 87–9.

12 Career Development Unit (CDU). www.oxforddeanerycdu.org.uk/about/about_cdu.html [accessed 25 June 2014].

MENTORING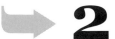

"Any drama?"

Dr Ted Sever, the on-take 9 p.m. ward round

___ Introduction

There are many definitions of mentoring, each focusing on different aspects of the role of mentor. Essentially, mentoring is a process of providing support, advice, knowledge and wisdom for the benefit of another individual (a mentee). A mentor helps another person through times of transition or changes in his or her personal circumstances.

The Standing Committee on Postgraduate Medical Education defines mentoring as a process whereby an experienced, highly regarded person (the mentor) guides another individual (the mentee) in the development of his or her own ideas, learning, and personal and professional development.[1]

Although mentoring is a dynamic relationship that is ever developing, it is important that the mentor and mentee are clear about what mentoring is in their particular context.[2]

___ History

Odysseus, before departing for the Trojan Wars, entrusted his friend Mentor with the responsibility of looking after his son Telemachus while he was away on his voyages. Odysseus was concerned that his son should develop the appropriate spiritual and personal values. Medieval mentoring related more to the craftsman–apprentice relationship. Present-day concepts of mentoring were revived in the United States in the 1970s, when mentoring became fashionable in corporate management. Managers would identify individuals with potential and fast-track them to senior positions.

Later mentoring became more popular in nurse education in helping student nurses make the transition from the lecture hall to the ward.[3]

Medical mentoring is not a management tool but is closely linked to the role of a teacher. The concept of mentoring seems to have moved from career development to tutor and role model and has now come full circle to the classical Homeric tradition of friend and supporter, a model that is adopted in this book.[4] A more modern fictional example of mentoring might be Obi-Wan Kenobi in the Star Wars films who was a mentor for Anakin Skywalker, with somewhat mixed results.[5]

___ Why have a mentor?

Students and doctors face major challenges in the course of their careers. The long career trajectory from school, through university and specialty training, to become an independent general practitioner can result in stress and in some cases burnout. Individuals need guidance and encouragement through these transitions if they are to become capable, competent and compassionate practitioners.[2]

Mentoring helps individuals through these transitions and may have further benefits in identifying potential and encouraging learners to develop. Mentors work right across the spectrum from high-flyers to those who are struggling, and including ethnic minorities and disadvantaged individuals. Mentors also play a part in stopping harassment and bullying.

Mentoring can develop professional attributes and facilitate socialisation into a profession.[6]

Mentoring can also play a part in supporting established general practitioners who may be at risk of compassion fatigue and burnout later in their careers. Indeed, while promoting individual self-development is the core of mentoring, its suggestions for change can have an impact on the organisational culture so that supporting staff is seen to be essential by the organisation.

Stenfors-Hayes *et al.* suggest that there are three ways of being a mentor:[7]

1_ By answering questions and giving advice

2_ By showing what it means to be a doctor, i.e. by acting as a role model

3_ By listening and stimulating reflection.

Being a mentor means supporting mentees' learning, preparing them for professional practice and inspiring them to be competent and compassionate doctors. A mentor must be interested and involved in the mentee's progress. He or she must be ready to adopt a number of different roles in response to the problems presented by the individual at a particular time.

These roles are summarised in Box 2.1 and explored in further detail later.

Box 2.1 **Roles of a mentor**

- Sounding-board.
- Adviser.
- Referee.
- Colleague.
- Networker.
- Confidante.
- Supporter.

- Empathiser.
- Coach.
- Advocate.
- Critical friend.
- Problem solver.
- Mirror.
- Role model.

___ Aims of mentoring

The work of the mentor is part of the teaching and support a student or trainee receives from a large number of staff. The mentor aims to help with anything that is impairing a student's or trainee's academic progress or a GP's performance. He or she assists in reducing stress, encourages lifelong reflective learning and makes education an enjoyable experience. Part of improving the performance of students and trainees is helping them to reflect on their work: they must be ready to identify what is going well and to recognise when they are not working well. This process of reflection is central to their learning and the mentor can show how it is not a boring tick-box exercise but part of becoming a mindful doctor. Giving constructive feedback to mentees is another core role of a mentor; the mentor can help to build self-confidence and encourage humility. Medicine is a complex, uncertain discipline and mistakes are bound to happen. Mentoring can assist mentees to learn from their mistakes and to seek to support colleagues who are having difficulties. In this way students and trainees learn effective multidisciplinary teamwork in which all colleagues, from all disciplines, are treated with respect and kindness.

___ Qualities of a mentor

Mentoring takes many forms but all those involved in supporting students and trainees share certain qualities (as shown on Table 2.1).

Table 2.1 **Qualities of a mentor**

Patience	Struggling students and trainees may be inconsistent in their behaviour, late for appointments and may not reply to emails. A mentor needs to work with these frustrations in helping the mentee with his or her problem
Confidence	The mentor should act as a role model and have a positive outlook
Competence	The clinician should be competent in his or her specialty and have credibility with colleagues
Commitment	The mentor must maintain interest over time to help students, trainees and colleagues
Integrity	The mentor should exhibit high standards of professional behaviour
Kindness	The mentor should be kind and approachable, recognising that it might have taken a great deal of courage for the troubled individual to come forward
Coach	The mentor must be competent enough to help teach the mentee in clinical skills and to help develop effective learning styles and exam technique
Humour	Learning should be fun and mentees and their mentors should be able to laugh at times and not take themselves too seriously
Humility	Medicine is a humbling discipline and humility a necessary virtue for being a doctor
Counsellor	Mentors should have good communication skills to give mentees the opportunity to talk about their difficulties
Organiser	To schedule meetings, keep records, manage time and plan

___ What to consider before taking on a mentor role

Anyone considering becoming a mentor should reflect on the following points before taking on the role.

Have I the time to take this on?

Mentees should be seen on average about twice a year and each meeting can last up to an hour. Reading essays, case discussions or portfolios also takes some time. Problems crop up and a student or doctor in difficulties will need more frequent meetings. Most meetings are initiated by the mentee and usually require a prompt response.

Have I the commitment to students and doctors to perform the role?

Struggling students and doctors may not answer emails, may forget appointments and may sometimes be angry and resentful. Mentors need patience and an ability to see this behaviour as part of the problem and not to react with immediate criticism. Mentees who have had a negative experience with a mentor will often be reluctant to consider contacting him or her for support in future. It can be helpful to keep in mind that every student and doctor was an 'A' student when they entered medical school.

Am I prepared to act as an advocate for the mentee?

At times a student may ask a mentor to plead his or her case to members of the medical school, which may involve the Academic Review Committee or discussion with senior colleagues. In cases of bullying or harassment the mentor may support the student or doctor during formal hearings. Although discussions with the mentee are confidential, there are rare instances when a person's behaviour puts patients at risk or the person is a risk to him or herself. In these rare situations the mentor has to warn the mentee that he or she has to inform the appropriate authority.

What are my own strengths and weaknesses?

Some of the qualities required to be a mentor were discussed earlier in this chapter. Many mentees are worried that having personal problems will be viewed negatively and may affect their career prospects. Mentors need to make it clear that the welfare of the mentee is their primary concern and that the individual has taken the right step in coming for help, and that this will have no deleterious effect on his or her record.

Do I need to learn any new skills?

New mentors might feel they need further training in certain areas, for example in giving feedback in a constructive way.

____ Choosing a mentor

In advising students, trainees or GPs on choosing a mentor it is helpful for them to reflect on the following questions:[8, 9]

- who takes an interest in your progress?
- who encourages you?
- who is a good role model?
- who has helped you in the past?
- who has challenged you to improve your practice?
- who is accessible and friendly?
- what is it about these people that has helped you?

A mentor should be enthusiastic and have a strong commitment to teaching and learning. A good listener, he or she should be sensitive to the needs of trainees. While every doctor should have a mentor, however, not every doctor is suitable to be one.[8]

A mentor must have empathy with the doctor and they need to agree boundaries to their relationship. They need to have realistic expectations of each other; a mentor cannot solve every problem but he or she can provide the time and space to address the issues. Perhaps simply giving a doctor in difficulty permission to raise his or her issues is one of the most useful functions of a mentor. Mentoring is an evolving relationship that is both supportive and challenging, and it must be confidential. Some personal issues may remain 'off the record', unless issues of patient safety arise. These boundaries must be made explicit from the outset. Mentors need to be skilled at providing feedback, an issue that is examined in detail in Chapter 5. Mentors should also know when they need to ask for help and when to refer a trainee to others.

____ How should mentoring take place?

What to do before a meeting

The mentor should book a mutually convenient time for the meeting. Communicating with a student, trainee or GP who also has fixed commitments and a variable timetable may require patience. Initial emails should be worded in a friendly manner, perhaps using given names. There has to be privacy for the one-to one meeting; confidentiality is crucial and a quiet setting conveys this to the mentee. It may be necessary to gather background information from a referring colleague before the meeting.

What to do during the meeting

Case story Nitin

Nitin is a fourth-year student noted as having no previous problems. He emails his mentor to ask for a meeting because he has just failed his end-of-year OSCE exam. Setting aside an hour, the mentor arranges to have a meeting in a quiet room where they will not be disturbed.

The mentor starts by welcoming Nitin and saying that she is pleased he has come and is sorry to hear that he has failed his exam. The mentor explains that she is not involved in his assessment, that her role is solely to help him and that the meeting is confidential.

Nitin looks downcast and is near to tears. The mentor empathises and reassures him that he can take his time just to explain how things went. He tells you that he failed two stations, in communication and in paediatrics. The mentor prompts him to reflect on stations that went well and points out that, even with the two stations where he scored badly, he only failed to pass by a narrow margin.

The mentor asks Nitin to describe what exactly happened in the two stations. He explains that in the communication station he had to counsel a 16-year-old girl in A&E who was requesting the 'morning after pill'.

With the mentor's prompting, Nitin says he covered the various choices open to the patient quite well. He then says that he totally ignored her emotional distress and had kept a rather distant 'professional' manner throughout.

The mentor asks why he did this and Nitin explains that he felt a bit flustered and embarrassed himself, and did not want to open an emotional 'can of worms' in a time-limited OSCE. The mentor finds out that in the ward situation Nitin is reported to have excellent communication skills and is comfortable discussing emotional issues with patients.

The mentor then asks about the specifics of the paediatric station. Nitin was asked about a baby's growth chart and, because he had not been on his paediatric ward for almost a year, had become confused and failed to spot that the baby was failing to thrive.

Yet again the mentor reminds Nitin that he did very well in several stations in the rest of the OSCE and in fact only marginally failed to gain a pass mark. The mentor asks him if there are any other difficulties with the course that concern him.

He is worried that this failure will count against him gaining a Foundation Year post. He says there is some tension with the landlord of his student flat who will not arrange plumbing repairs. He asks for help in improving his performance in the resit OSCE.

The mentor reassures Nitin that he is a good student and that he is going to qualify and get a Foundation post. She explains that many students slip up in an occasional exam but it is always more of a fright when it occurs late in the course for the first

23

time. She suggests that a practice session of OSCE communication stations might help to restore his confidence. Nitin is keen on this idea and the mentor fixes a slot for him with a clinical tutor in a couple of weeks' time.

The mentor asks if he would like to attend the paediatric ward for some extra sessions and offers to speak to a registrar she knows who can arrange this with Nitin.

She also gives him the number of student accommodation services. They may be able to help with his landlord problem.

The mentor arranges to see Nitin in a month and encourages him to keep in touch by email.

....

Note: Nitin attends the OSCE revision session and the extra work on the paediatric ward. He passes his resit easily and is now a Foundation Doctor with plans for a career in chest medicine.

Structure of the meeting: ten tips

From the case study of a struggling student the following ten tips emerge:

1_ Introductions

2_ Put the individual at ease and reassure him or her that the meeting is confidential. Explain that your role is supportive and you are pleased that he or she has come for help. Identify the purpose of the meeting and be clear about the mentee's expectations

3_ Explain that you will take notes and what will happen to the record

4_ Start by asking how things are going

5_ Explore work and study patterns

6_ Explore the specific issues raised by the mentee

7_ Discuss various solutions

8_ The mentee agrees on an action plan

9_ Offer continuing support and give contact details

10_ Arrange follow-up.

___ Follow-up

As the mentee puts the agreed plan into action the cycle begins again, creating a learning spiral in which the mentee gains in self-awareness and deepens his or her understanding. The mentee moves from a position of dependence to become independent. At this stage the mentee is comfortable to be challenged about his or her views and to accept constructive criticism and feedback.

What to do after the meeting

- Document the meeting.
- Pass on any conclusions that the mentee has agreed might be put in his or her file.
- Consider referral.
- Make sure you implement any tasks you have agreed to carry out.

When to refer

Individuals who might benefit from more specialist help should, with their consent, be referred to the appropriate service. The medical school or General Medical Council (GMC) should be notified if there is a question of the student's fitness to practise.

___ Personal tutor support and networking

A mentor can provide help both for mentees and their personal tutors by establishing a good working relationship with tutors. He or she must be ready to accept referred students. For example, it can be useful, with a student's consent, to brief a block supervisor of a student's recent bereavement. Personal tutors can also discuss any student who is causing concern with the mentor so that support may be provided before any possible exam failure. Small group tutorials offering practical tips for new tutors are an opportunity both to address tutors' concerns and to provide training in supporting students and trainees.

___ Organising a mentoring system

The organisation must believe in the value of mentoring and be prepared to demonstrate its commitment. Managers should raise awareness of the mentoring system and be clear about the aims and outcomes of mentoring. They should ensure that the mentoring ethos is consistent with their own culture within the organisation. The organisation needs to be aware of the identity of the mentors and mentees with whom it is involved. Mentors require training and support, and there should be some evaluation of the mentoring system. Optimally the mentees should be able to choose their mentor but this may not always be practical.

There is a great potential for developing mentoring schemes in the NHS. Referral for a mentor's support should follow any investigation of concerns about a doctor's professional competency. There is a need to achieve a more appropriate balance between regulation and support by organisations such as the GMC and the National Clinical Assessment Service (NCAS).

Benefits of mentoring

Mentoring can benefit the mentee, the mentor and the organisation.

MENTEE

Mentees gets a listening ear, valuable direction, gaps filled in, doors opened and a different perspective on their problems. They may also gain greater self-confidence and be able to develop their reflective learning skills. They should become more comfortable about accepting praise and criticism. Mentees may become more politically aware and gain increased understanding of their organisation. They will feel supported through transition times, developing a broader outlook, becoming more able to embrace change and willing to take risks. Job satisfaction will be increased and they will have a better sense of the direction of their career path. Increasingly sensitive to the needs of colleagues, mentees will have improved team-working skills. They can also benefit from one-to-one teaching and encouragement to reflect on their learning experiences.[2]

General practitioners can benefit from mentoring in three areas: their professional practice, personal wellbeing and their professional development.[10] The benefits extend beyond the doctor's professional role and cross the professional–personal interface.[10] Mentoring seems to have most effect on problem solving and change management but the benefits are not restricted to one domain. Many doctors come to mentoring when their self-confidence is low as a result of workload pressures, difficult relationships with colleagues, personal problems and feeling undervalued by their colleagues.[10] Mentoring can help to restore self-confidence by suggesting fresh ways of tackling problems. Many doctors need help with problems arising at the professional–personal interface: relationships, job satisfaction, performance, managing change and problem solving. Job satisfaction and a sense of belonging to a medical community can be increased by mentoring.[10] Other problems that may be encountered by general practitioners relate to: practice re-organisation, service delivery, home–work balance, changing jobs, career development, complaints and disciplinary procedures.[10]

MENTOR

Mentors will gain in self-awareness and will develop their skills in giving and receiving feedback. There is a strong link between mentoring and teaching. Mentoring involves reflecting on one's own values.[11] Mentoring involves keeping up to date in knowledge and being familiar with the curriculum and organisation. Contact with colleagues brings opportunities for giving and receiving support. Increased job satisfaction comes with the feeling that one is helping colleagues to flourish and achieve their potential. Passing on one's experience is rewarding in itself. Negotiating skills are improved as one develops the ability to encourage, challenge and support others.

ORGANISATION

The benefits of mentoring extend beyond the doctor's professional role. The organisation benefits by having staff who feel valued and supported. Access to mentoring improves morale, staff retention and recruitment, and there is less burnout. Mentoring fosters a culture of trust and confidentiality, and as a result team-working is improved.[2]

It is likely that NHS organisations would be improved by doctors who feel valued and more fulfilled in their professional roles as a result of mentoring.[10] Patients benefit by the improved professional practice, team-working and increased confidence of doctors who receive mentoring.[10] There is now official support for mentoring of NHS doctors from the Royal College of General Practitioners.[12]

___ Conclusion

This chapter introduced mentoring. In the next chapter the mentoring relationship is explored in much greater depth.

Key points

Mentoring is supportive.

Mentors share certain personal qualities.

Should I become a mentor?

How to choose a mentor.

How to structure a meeting with your mentee.

Mentoring has benefits to the mentee, the NHS and to patients.

___ References

1 Standing Committee on Postgraduate Medical Education. *Supporting Doctors and Dentists at Work: an enquiry into mentoring.* London: SCOPME, 1998.

2 McKimm J, Jollie C, Hatter M, London Deanery. *Mentoring: theory and practice.* London: Faculty Development, www.faculty.londondeanery.ac.uk/e-learning/feedback/files/Mentoring_Theory_and_Practice.pdf [accessed 25 June 2014].

3 Andrews M, Wallis M. Mentorship in nursing: a literature review. *Journal of Advanced Nursing* 1999; **29(1)**: 201–7.

4 Bulstrode C, Hunt V. What is mentoring? *Lancet* 2000; **356(9244)**: 1788.

5 Star Wars. http://starwars.com/explore/the-movies/episode-iii/ [accessed 25 June 2014].

6 Kalen S, Stenfors-Hayes T, Hylin U, *et al.* Mentoring medical students during classroom courses: a way to enhance professional development. *Medical Teacher* 2010; **32(8)**: 315–21.

7 Stenfors-Hayes T, Hult H, Dahlgren LO. What does it mean to be a mentor in medical education? *Medical Teacher* 2011; **33(8)**: 423–8.

8 Cooper N, Forrest K. *Essential Guide to Educational Supervision in Postgraduate Medical Education.* London: BMJ Books, Wiley-Blackwell, 2009.

9 Gupta RC, Lingam S. *Mentoring for Doctors and Dentists.* Oxford: Blackwell Science, 2000.

10 Steven A, Oxley J, Fleming W G. Mentoring for NHS doctors: perceived benefits across the personal-professional interface. *Journal of the Royal Society of Medicine* 2008; **101(11)**: 552–7.

11 Stenfors-Hayes T, Kalen S, Hult H, *et al.* Being a mentor for undergraduate medical students enhances personal and professional development. *Medical Teacher* 2010; **32(2)**: 148–53.

12 Royal College of General Practitioners. *Teaching, Mentoring and Clinical Supervision.* Curriculum Statement 3.7. London: RCGP, 2007, www.rcgp.org.uk/gp-training-and-exams/gp-curriculum-overview/gp-curriculum-previous-versions.aspx [accessed 25 June 2014].

THE MENTORING RELATIONSHIP 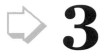 3

Listen
Dr M.R. Rajagopal, a sign on the wall in the palliative care clinic in Calicut

___ Introduction

In this chapter the mentoring relationship is explored, beginning by looking at what students and doctors in training expect from a mentor.[1]

___ What do mentees want?

What do struggling students value in a mentor?

Accessibility

Sometimes students report difficulty in establishing relationships with mentors. Face-to-face contact is often limited and students may feel intimidated when contacting a busy senior clinician. Students are far more likely to trust mentors with whom they have a regular contact than those to whom they are referred when they have failed an exam.

Respecting confidentiality

A respect for confidentiality is essential in a successful student–mentor relationship. Although students are generally happy to approach staff about academic matters, they are less sure about contacting mentors about personal issues. Confidentiality is important on both sides.

Giving feedback

Students prefer face-to-face feedback; it is valuable to meet a mentor on a regular basis to discuss his or her understanding of the curriculum. Giving some positive feedback builds self-confidence and helps students to address deficiencies.

Knowledge of curriculum

Students value support from staff who have an understanding of the medical curriculum and know what is expected of the student at each stage. Mentors who can draw on their own experiences at medical school are better equipped to relate to a student's particular situation. Mentors can provide insights into the medical profession and the rites and customs related to medicine: the 'hidden curriculum'.

Academic guidance

It may be possible for mentors to help students identify educational needs and to advise them about effective learning strategies. Mentors can help students by giving feedback on their clinical case discussions or on their clinical portfolios. Students may need help and encouragement to use reflection as an aid to learning.

Professional development

Role modelling is a powerful learning tool. Mentors have opportunities to be good role models by demonstrating openness to discussing their strengths and weaknesses. By modelling the reflective process and how this improves clinical practice, mentors can enhance the students' own professional development.

Knowledge of sources of support available

Students benefit from mentors who are well informed of the range of available support and when to make referral to other agencies.

Respect, empathy and patience

Students who are struggling need encouragement and sometimes consoling. Some students, having never failed an exam before, find the experience devastating, with a consequent loss of confidence. It is surprising that some students seem to lose confidence as the course progresses and may even doubt that they wish to continue in medicine.

Personal support

Mentors should possess the counselling skills to respond sensitively to students who experience a range of personal problems. There may be family problems with a breakdown of relationships causing mental anguish. Depression may occur and present in failing exams or unexplained absences. Financial worries about funding their course may be difficult for students to discuss. Stress from their workload or from exam anxiety can impair performance in assessments. Once students are confident that they can trust the mentor they then disclose these personal concerns.

Advocacy

Mentors may be required to act as an advocate for the student. Sometimes this may create a conflict of interest and then further advice should be sought. Where the mentor is required to write a report on the student's progress, consent must be given.

Career advice

Where students need information about specific career paths the mentor should be able to provide suitable contacts. The university career service may also give individual help on career choices, interview techniques and writing a CV.

___ Doctors in training

Goodyear *et al.* found that Foundation Year doctors had equivocal experiences of mentoring during their undergraduate training.[2] Most of the doctors wanted a mentor but said they would prefer to choose one. The top five characteristics of good mentoring were: being supportive, ensuring confidentiality, providing feedback, being honest and having good listening skills. The doctors were confused about the distinction between an educational supervisor and a mentor. The Foundation doctors looked to the mentor for career advice and advice about specialist training, motivation, help with clinical problems, a sounding board, emotional support and networking.[2] Lloyd and Becker reported that paediatric specialist registrars valued feedback on their performance, career advice and objective setting from their educational supervisors. In this paper they commented that poor aspects of supervision were a lack of commitment, talking rather than listening and a need for more encouragement.[3]

___ The relationship

The mentees discussed in this book – students, trainees and general practitioners – are colleagues not patients. When mentors are in their clinical role they adopt a range of sophisticated communication skills, emotions, attitudes and competencies for the benefit of the patient. A mentoring model can be designed that utilises these same skills, knowledge and attitudes for the benefit of students and doctors. The skills involved cover such areas as: taking a careful history, identifying the struggling student or doctor in difficulty and gathering further information. They also include: making a diagnosis, negotiating a management plan with the mentee, knowing when to refer for help and arranging follow-up to provide continuity of care.[4] Just as in the clinical situation where patients present with a complex combination of physical, psychological and social problems, students and doctors also have complex factors interacting to affect their performance.

Confidentiality and trust form the foundation of the doctor–patient relationship and they are equally important in the mentor–mentee relationship. However, it is vital that the mentor needs to appreciate that he or she is not the mentee's doctor. This aspect of the relationship will be discussed further in this chapter.

Every student, trainee and general practitioner should have a mentor, particularly at the transition points in their careers, which have been discussed. Mentoring should be available for all medical students and doctors, not just those who have been identified as struggling. Clinical teachers are ideally placed to act as mentors and are in the best position to identify early signs of a student or doctor having difficulty. If supportive interventions can be introduced early then major problems may be avoided.[5]

Mentors need to have the skills to recognise the signs of a student or doctor in difficulty (Chapter 4). They need diagnostic skills to clarify the problems and therapeutic skills to discuss and agree a plan of management with the student or doctor.[4] A patient-centred interviewing model to guide the discussion with the mentee follows both strands clinicians use in their consultation with patients.[4,6] One strand follows a biomedical model that focuses on the disease and traditionally involves taking a history, carrying out an examination, arranging investigations and so reaching a differential diagnosis. The other strand follows the patient's agenda and is focused on the broader concept of the meaning of the illness to the patient. This strand involves exploring the patient's Ideas, Concerns and Expectations about his or her illness and the impact it has on the patient's life. The outcome is a shared understanding of the situation between the patient and doctor. Normally these two strands to the consultation are integrated in a patient-centred approach.[4]

In a mentee-centred approach, the agenda of the mentor that might be focused on exam results, revalidation reports, attendance or performance issues is integrated with the mentee's agenda. This may be focused on partnership problems, family issues, stress or a lack of motivation.[4] A skilled mentor will follow the student's or doctor's agenda, exploring his or her Ideas, Concerns and Expectations before introducing discussion of the mentee's agenda, which might include an issue affecting performance. Too often the mentee's agenda is left to the end of the interview or is neglected altogether.

Just as the results of investigations can contribute to a patient's care so too can objective data on the student or trainee help in discussions. This data might be an exam result, feedback from colleagues or attendance records. These results may back up impressions gained from the history.

In devising a way forward to help the student or trainee, the mentor can use the same therapeutic skills that he or she uses in negotiating a management plan with the patient. In a mentee-centred approach the student or trainee comes to recognise, acknowledge and deal with the issues affecting their performance.[4]

However, in adopting an open mentee-centred approach the mentor may fear that he or she is going to 'open a can of worms'. Some clinicians distance themselves from patients for the same reason. However, if the mentor is to have a trusting relationship with the mentee he or she must give the individual an opportunity to discuss real concerns. The foundation of effective personal support is empathy, both in a clinical consultation and in mentoring.[7]

Supporting a struggling student or doctor in many ways mirrors the clinical consultation, but the focus of care and attention is a mentee not a patient. Supporting students and trainees involves adopting an empathic role, attempting to see the world through their eyes. The aim of a meeting is to provide a supportive, confidential environment in which the mentee is able to voice his or her concerns. This can be helped by agreeing ground rules at the outset.

___ Ground rules for mentor meetings

- Confidentiality.

- Time out – the mentee has control over answering questions or to stop if distressed.

- Honesty.

- Non-judgemental.

- Non-threatening.

- Open to the possibility of change.

- Respect for each other.

- Don't take yourself too seriously. Both mentee and mentor may need to 'lighten up'.

Both parties need to be clear about their own expectations of the meeting. They need to agree on the level of formality, methods of communication and frequency of meetings. After discussion, the mentee should feel empowered to make his or her own decision on an agreed plan of action.

Boundaries

The mentor should respect boundaries and not over-identify with the mentee. The mentee may only want a listening ear, not an instant solution. There should be a readiness to refer when the mentee needs further help. The problems that may occur in relation to boundaries are discussed in Chapter 12.

Counselling skills

Mentoring is not counselling but, as in clinical practice, counselling skills are required. These include building rapport, drawing the trainee out with open questions and managing silence to listen deeply. The mentor should then be able to check with the mentee that he or she has a correct understanding of the problem. Further time is given to clarifying and summarising the issue, and by the end of this process the mentor and mentee set objectives and arrange the follow-up. Allowing the mentee time and space gives him or her permission to raise difficult problems.

Challenge

Mentoring relationships based on support sometimes also need to challenge the mentee so that he or she grows professionally. The two elements of support and challenge must be combined because, if the mentor simply challenges a mentee without support and trust, the mentee will simply regress in his or her professional development. Effective mentors combine support and challenge by providing opportunities and setting positive expectations.[8]

Empathy

Goldie describes empathy as a process by which a person imagines the narrative (thoughts, feelings and emotions) of another person. Empathy is an imaginative process that results in us having the same type of feeling or emotions as other people. There are three components of empathy:[9, 10]

1_ Affective matching – the mentor experiences the same emotions as the mentee

2_ Other-orientated perspective taking – I imagine that I am you in your situation. I try to simulate your experience from your point of view. This can be contrasted with self-orientated perspective taking where I imagine what it is like for me to be in your situation. One of the useful products of this self–other differentiation in perspective taking is that it stops us assuming that we understand the other person's experience when we do not. Empathy is a unique kind of understanding through which we can come close to experiencing what it is like to be another person. Rather than trying to understand the other person from some distant objective perspective we try to share the other person's perspective[10]

3_ Self–other differentiation – it is essential to retain an awareness of the other as another individual to avoid becoming too involved with him or her. We need to achieve the optimal level of distance to allow for deep engagement and successful empathy without being damaged by the process.[10]

___ The mentor–mentee relationship

As the mentor and mentee connect at a deeper level, the relationship develops; the mentor can be more challenging because a mentee may benefit from being taken out of his or her comfort zone. This gives them a chance to explore possibilities 'off the record' and may result in ideas that change their practice. Formal records must be kept of professional issues and the mentee should see these and agree them. Personal issues may be kept entirely confidential with no record being made provided that there is no patient safety consideration. Mentors must be ready to follow their own advice that they give to their mentees and to seek help from a senior colleague if there is a confidentiality issue.

Facilitating the personal and professional development of the mentee lies at the heart of mentoring.[11] The mentor should have belief in their mentees, that they are bright and are keen to learn. Mentoring values the diversity between individuals and their learning styles. Mentors should encourage a sense of curiosity in the mentee, fostering collaboration not competition. In developing reflective skills the mentor facilitates the mentee to have the capability to transfer learning to new situations.

Mentoring individuals through times of transition involves giving them space to develop their professional competency and gives them a sense of belonging to a community as they are acknowledged as colleagues.[12] Mentoring can encourage the student or trainee to have greater self-confidence and motivation. By demonstrating empathy the mentor can enable the mentee to learn from emotional experiences and to be prepared to change. A mentor can generate a sense of security even in uncertain situations, mirroring the feeling of safety that a patient feels in the hands of a caring doctor or nurse. Giving a mentee a sense of security can increase motivation and generate hope.

The mentor–mentee relationship is, like the doctor–patient relationship, a special relationship. The two people involved make a real connection with each other and form a bond.[13] It is in this one-to-one relationship that the student or doctor can develop reflective capacity, empathy and a sense of belonging to a professional community.[12] Mentors bring experience and wisdom to setting the mentee's problems in a wider context. Giving mentees space to reflect on their performance without being judgemental allows them to share their doubts and feelings.

The mentor relationship develops and changes over time. At first the mentor provides a safe, protected environment that enables him or her to be a supporter and guide. As the mentee develops self-confidence and becomes less dependent, mentoring can take on a more analytical, challenging and reflective role to enhance deep learning.[13] The quality of this relationship, like the quality of the doctor–patient relationship, determines the success of the outcome. Mentor and mentee should have an equal relationship where dependency is not encouraged. Both partners should be comfortable in giving and receiving honest feedback.

Young doctors found it helpful when mentors shared their own mistakes and vulnerabilities.[14] Mentoring also depends upon continuity, as it is an evolving relationship of trust. It provides a forum where both pastoral and educational issues can be discussed. Mentoring does not involve assessment and is therefore non-threatening, allowing GPs to discuss their problems without losing face. Thus mentors need to be non-judgemental and also have experience of medical education, practice administration and politics.[14] Mentors should not impose their agenda on their mentees. Mentoring establishes a culture where sensitive issues can be raised and vulnerabilities discussed. It should not be reserved for doctors in difficulty but should be available to all doctors. It is much easier and less time consuming to prevent stress and burnout than to deal with the consequences.[14]

___ Listening to the story

In clinical practice doctors commonly interrupt patients before they can tell their story. On average a doctor will interrupt only 17 seconds after the patient starts talking. It is interesting to observe that if patients are allowed to talk without interruption they will usually finish speaking in 90 seconds. If doctors interrupt patients they will miss over half the patient's concerns.[15, 16]

Deep listening is listening not just to the content of the patient's words but also listening to discover the meaning behind the patient's words. Listening in this attentive way involves checking with the patient that both parties have a clear understanding of what has been said. This applies in exactly the same way in the mentor–mentee relationship. Deep listening is not just an attempt to understand communication but it is a form of empathy, i.e. to experience what it is to be the other person. Attention to non-verbal communication, body language and the use of silence enables the doctor and the mentor to listen deeply. This form of relationship is therapeutic in itself.[15]

The mentor should use his or her communication skills of listening, questioning, clarifying and reflecting to hear the mentee's story. In analysing the information and then reflecting on possible ways forward, the model of Johari's window may be useful.[13]

Figure 3.1 **Johari's window**

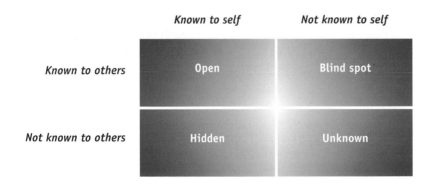

<table>
<tr><td></td><td>*Known to self*</td><td>*Not known to self*</td></tr>
<tr><td>*Known to others*</td><td>Open</td><td>Blind spot</td></tr>
<tr><td>*Not known to others*</td><td>Hidden</td><td>Unknown</td></tr>
</table>

An individual's ability to develop, share information and deepen awareness is determined by his or her self-awareness and by how much an individual decides to reveal about him or herself. Using the Johari model, an individual can develop self-awareness by seeking feedback and reducing his or her 'blind spot'. He or she can also contribute to the mentoring relationship by disclosure and so reducing the 'hidden' area.[13]

Mentoring is a flexible concept that can be modified to suit particular individuals or the requirements of the workplace. Most commonly it is a one-to-one relationship but mentoring can take place in groups. In some situations peer-mentoring works well. A mentor can provide continuity and support for young doctors, who may feel anonymous on different wards where they meet many different clinicians for short periods of time.

___ Managing change

Mentors may find the Stages of Change model helpful in their motivational interviewing. This breaks the process of change in behaviour into stages and thus change becomes less daunting for the mentee. It is also helpful for the mentor to have realistic goals for each meeting.[17]

At first, in the Precontemplation phase, the mentee is unaware that there is a problem. At this stage the mentor's task is to raise awareness by giving feedback.

> *For instance, Becky, a trainee, might not realise how irritating it is for patients and practice staff if she always starts her surgeries five minutes late.*

In the next stage of Contemplation the mentee becomes aware of the problem but as yet has done nothing to change it.

> *At this stage Becky becomes aware that always being late is unprofessional and discourteous to others, and shows a lack of respect for other people.*

In the Preparation phase the person makes adjustments to make the change.

> *Becky asks her child minder to arrive half an hour earlier in the mornings.*

In the Action phase the mentee makes the necessary changes to their behaviour.

Becky arrives 15 minutes before surgery, spends some time greeting the reception staff and her colleagues, and is prepared to see her first patient on time.

In the Maintenance phase the mentor gives feedback on the effects of the change.

The mentor tells Becky how much happier the staff are and there have been positive comments from patients.

While motivating the mentee to make a change in some aspect of his or her behaviour, the mentor needs to be encouraging and non-judgemental. The mentor must allow time for the mentee to express negative emotions. This facilitates the development of mutual trust and allows the mentee to develop the self-confidence to make the change.[15, 18]

___ Conclusion

The mentor should be able to help with the 'hidden curriculum': ethics, attitudes and professionalism. He or she must have knowledge of the curriculum, clinical competency and an interest in the mentee's welfare. As mentoring is a reciprocal relationship, mentors can share their own vulnerabilities and in doing so the mentee learns of the uncertainties and dilemmas that are a part of clinical practice. While being aware of the risk of dependency, an enthusiastic mentor can inspire a mentee to be self-directed in his or her learning.

There are many different ways of mentoring; the Homeric view is of a wise counsellor, trusted friend and role model. Modern mentors have been described as critical friends.[7] Most models describe a one-to-one relationship but group mentoring, peer mentoring and e-mentoring are alternative approaches. People often form mentor-like relationships outside of any formal mentoring framework as mentoring is a relationship not a management activity. Informal mentoring can work but depends on the right people finding each other.[19]

Mentoring works best when the mentee has a choice of mentor because compatibility is key to the trusting relationship. The relationship that may start with an emphasis on support and guidance changes as the mentee develops confidence, and the mentor can become more challenging, critical and reflective while still being supportive and encouraging.

In this type of relationship, based on empathy and honesty, the mentor can give a broader perspective of the profession and set the issues in a sensible perspective. By sharing their experience and expertise the mentor helps the mentee to achieve his or her goals.[20]

Key points

Students and doctors need encouragement.

Listening not interrupting.

Empathy is at the heart of mentoring.

A clinical model may be adapted to mentoring.

Mentoring can motivate change.

—— References

1 Robertson F, Donaldson C, Jarvis R, Jeffrey D. How can an academic mentor improve support of tomorrow's doctors? *Scottish Universities Medical Journal* 2013: **2(2)**: 28–38.

2 Goodyear H, Bindal N, Bindal T, Wall D. Foundation doctors' experiences and views of mentoring. *British Journal of Hospital Medicine* 2013; **74(12)**: 682–6.

3 Lloyd B, Becker D. Paediatric specialist registrars' views on educational supervision and how it can be improved. *Journal of the Royal Society of Medicine* 2007; **100(8)**: 375–8.

4 Evans D E, Alstead E M, Brown J. Applying your clinical skills to students and trainees in academic difficulty. *The Clinical Teacher* 2010; **7(4)**: 230–5.

5 Evans D, Brown J. Supporting students in difficulty. In: P Cantillon, D Woods (eds), *ABC of Learning and Teaching in Medicine*. Chichester: Wiley-Blackwell, 2010, pp. 78–82.

6 Levenstein J H, McCracken E C, McWhinney I R, *et al*. The patient-centred clinical method 1. A model for the doctor-patient interaction in family medicine. *Family Practice* 1986; **3(1)**: 24–30.

7 Cooper N, Forrest K. *Essential Guide to Educational Supervision in Postgraduate Medical Education*. London: BMJ Books, Wiley-Blackwell, 2009.

8 Ramani S, Gruppen L, Kachur E K. Twelve tips for developing effective mentors. *Medical Teacher* 2006; **28(5)**: 404–8.

9 Matravers D. Empathy as a route to knowledge. In: A Coplan, P Goldie (eds), *Empathy: philosophical and psychological perspectives*. Oxford: Oxford University Press, 2011, pp. 19–30.

10 Coplan A. Understanding empathy. In: A Coplan, P Goldie (eds), *Empathy: philosophical and psychological perspectives*. Oxford: Oxford University Press, 2011, pp. 3–18.

11 Kalen S, Stenfors-Hayes T, Hylin U, *et al.* Mentoring medical students during clinical courses: a way to enhance professional development. *Medical Teacher* 2010: **32(8)**: 315–21.

12 Kalen S, Ponzer S, Silen C. The core of mentorship: medical students' experiences of one-to-one mentoring in a clinical environment. *Advances in Health Sciences Education: theory and practice* 2012; **17(3)**: 389–401.

13 McKimm J, Jollie C, Hatter M, London Deanery. *Mentoring: theory and practice.* London: Faculty Development, www.faculty.londondeanery.ac.uk/e-learning/feedback/files/Mentoring_Theory_and_Practice.pdf [accessed 25 June 2014].

14 Alliott R. Facilitatory mentoring in general practice. *BMJ Careers Focus* 1996; **313**: S2–7060.

15 Amery J. *The Integrated Practitioner: co-creating in health practice.* Oxford: Radcliffe Publishing, 2013.

16 Kurtz S M, Silverman J, Draper J. *Teaching and Learning Communication Skills in Medicine.* Oxford: Radcliffe Publishing, 2004.

17 Prochaska J O, DiClemente C C. *The Transtheoretical Approach: crossing traditional boundaries of therapy.* Melbourne, FL: R E Krieger, 1994.

18 Sandman L, Munthe C. Shared decision making, paternalism and patient choice. *Health Care Analysis* 2010; **18(1)**: 60–84.

19 Newcastle University. *Academic and Research Mentoring Scheme: guidance notes.* www.ncl.ac.uk/staffdev/assets/documents/mentoring-academicresearch-guidelines_aj.pdf [accessed 25 June 2014].

20 Hay J. *Transformational Mentoring.* New York: McGraw-Hill, 1995.

STUDENTS AND DOCTORS IN DIFFICULTY: TRANSITIONS 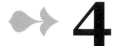 4

"Have you ever thought of specialising in palliative care?"
Dr Derek Doyle, on a visit to a patient's home

___ Introduction

Medical students, doctors in training and general practitioners may have a combination of problems that interact to cause them to struggle. All students and doctors want to be regarded as professionals with the highest standards but, nevertheless, every doctor has had to struggle at some stage in his or her career. Unfortunately, because of a general denial that doctors are vulnerable, most students and doctors feel that there is a stigma in seeking help. This may leave the individual feeling unsupported, isolated and stressed.

___ Medical students

The requirements of the formal curriculum can combine with the more subtle elements of the 'hidden curriculum' to cause stress, lowered self-confidence and impaired learning.[1]

Medical education contains three elements:

1_ Formal curriculum – laid out and lists what the student has to cover

2_ Informal curriculum – *ad hoc*, informal, interpersonal learning between staff and students

3_ Hidden curriculum – influences that are set at an organisational and cultural level.

Medical students undergo an arduous selection process. The student's personality can determine how he or she will fit in with the formal curriculum.[1] Incorporation into the medical community (hidden curriculum) also depends on a socialisation process that is influenced by the student's values and interpersonal interactions. Students may react to stress by coping or by showing some form of dysfunctional behaviour. How they react may depend on their vulnerability to dysfunctional behaviour. Dysfunctional tendencies may be triggered by stress and be shown in several ways: substance misuse, mental illness, sexual harassment and unethical behaviour.[1]

Academic workload is often the first stress encountered by students. They need to adjust learning styles to become deeper learners, take exams and face uncertainty. At this stage they encounter the first ritual in the informal curriculum, which is an accepted part of medical education but can be stressful.

Case story Cathy

Cathy bursts into tears on seeing a human cadaver. She has never seen a dead body before. Her grandfather died a year earlier while Cathy was on a gap year; she had missed his funeral and has felt guilty and sad since.

Dissection of a human cadaver is something of a rite of passage in many medical schools. Cathy's emotional reaction made her feel that she could never become a doctor. Some of her class also felt that her reaction showed that she was weak and probably not tough enough to finish her course. This stoical ethic and its underlying value of scientific detachment is part of the medical school culture.[1]

Medical students are subjected to various stresses in the informal curriculum. They can suffer humiliation in front of their colleagues and racial or sexual harassment. These abuses can result in the student becoming cynical, having decreased self-confidence, a reduced ability to learn or even leading to alcohol and substance misuse.[1]

Knights *et al.* carried out personality testing on medical students and found four categories of potentially dysfunctional traits:[1]

Tendency to move away from people – was associated with moodiness, detachment and independence, found in 23% of the students in their study. When stressed, these students have a tendency to be unpredictable and to overreact to criticism. They may be defensive, reluctant to try new methods, procrastinate, and prefer to work alone.

Tendency to move against people – these students were self-confident and were able to take risks. They were impulsive and not afraid of failure. Ten per cent of the students had high scores associated with aggressiveness, competitiveness and self-promotion.

Diligent – these students were characterised by a tendency to perfectionism. They were orderly and well-organised. However, those students with high scores, indicating dysfunctional traits, were liable to be pedantic, uncooperative, critical and stubborn. They created stress for themselves by trying to do too much and failing to delegate.

Dutiful – These students tended to be pleasant and friendly. They were good team players and were reluctant to express disagreement. But there was a tendency for students in the high range to be indecisive. They were too ready to rely on others to make decisions.

Transitions in the student's career can be the most troubled times. The list below includes some of the common reasons why students struggle. Most often there is a cluster of reasons why the person is in difficulty. Part of the skill in mentoring is listening, clarifying and defining the heart of the problem.

___ Reasons for struggling: medical students

Academic

Academic reasons for struggling include assessments and exams, resits, fear of failure, workload, negative feedback, uncertainty of what is expected of students, career prospects, study skills problems and time management.

Health

Health problems can be related to disability, dyslexia, chronic disease, alcohol, smoking or drug misuse.

Psychological

Mental health problems include depression, obsessive compulsive disorder, anxiety state, performance anxiety, social phobia and eating disorders. There are a variety of situations in which the student may feel stressed, for example seeing a dead body, human dissection, dealing with dying patients and managing acutely ill patients.

Social

Social problems may include family bereavement, relationship difficulties, clinical attachments away from university, dysfunctional tutorial groups, cultural issues, gender issues, language problems, racism, loneliness, financial pressures, bullying, family problems, adjusting to university life and accommodation issues.

One of the challenges facing a mentor is a student who has no insight into his or her problem. For instance, conscientiousness can slip into becoming perfectionism, where there is a failure to delegate. Students who lack insight fail to see the impact of their behaviour on those around them and so lack any motivation to change their behaviour or to seek help. Insight can prevent a student running into difficulty and also from being too bored or too stressed.

___ Reasons why doctors find themselves in difficulty

As discussed earlier, doctors are encouraged to adopt a stoical approach and not to admit to any weakness. They have had limited access to help and failing doctors may be ostracised and often opt for a different career.[2] More recently there has been a change of culture to try to identify such doctors and to provide them with support.

General practitioners identify stressors such as the demands of their job, patient expectations, practice administration, patient complaints, work–home balance and fear of assault.[3]

The National Clinical Assessment Service (NCAS) provides advice and support in managing poor performance and doctors in difficulty.[4] NCAS has devised a Performance Triangle to describe the reasons doctors are in difficulty (see Figure 4.1).

A question arises as to whether the problem is a doctor in difficulty or a difficult doctor. It may be hard to differentiate the factors concerned with the doctor's personality from issues of competence. NCAS found that in 1000 doctors referred to the service Behaviour (Misconduct) was a factor in 58% of cases, Health in 23% and Clinical concerns in 61%.[4]

Concerns are identified in a number of ways: appraisals and revalidation, complaints, corridor conversations and from the clinical governance systems.[4] Early warning signs of a doctor in difficulty are discussed later in this chapter. NCAS found that health concerns included physical health, mental health, stress, burnout and substance misuse. Misconduct included breach of contract, crime, fraud, sexual impropriety and inappropriate behaviour at work. They found that poor communication with colleagues was an issue more commonly than communication problems with patients.[4]

Figure 4.1 **NCAS Performance Triangle**

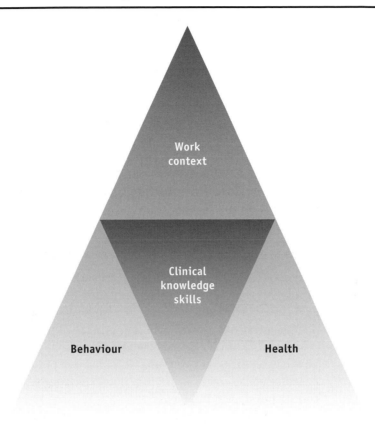

Source: McLaughlan C. *Managing Poor Performance and Doctors in Difficulty.*[4] Copyright© National Clinical Assessment Service. Used with permission.

—— Health problems

Doctors are poor at recognising their own health problems (see Chapter 9) and may be inhibited from seeking help if they are suffering from mental illness, fearing that they might be stigmatised. Young doctors are vulnerable to depression and alcohol misuse.[5] Doctors have higher rates of mental health problems, including alcohol and substance misuse, than the general population; they are also prone to depression and burnout.[6] Doctors often present late with high levels of distress and with severe problems, usually alcohol dependency and depression.[5] The severity of the problem at presentation may be due to the doctor delaying seeking help. It is common for doctors to treat themselves to avoid disclosing their health problems because they are concerned about breaches in confidentiality or the effect on their careers.

___ Work

General practitioners report finding the following most stressful: living with uncertainty, unresolved complaints, feelings of inadequacy and loss of control of their working lives.[7] Performance problems include poor judgement, a lack of knowledge and inadequate clinical skills. Some of these issues may be picked up in appraisals or during revalidation.

___ Behaviour

Behavioural problems may include rudeness, intolerance, lack of punctuality or angry outbursts. They may also involve even more serious breaches of professional conduct such as bullying, harassment, racism or inappropriate sexual behaviour towards patients or colleagues.

Bullying has been tolerated in the NHS in the past. Bullying causes doctors to lose confidence, feel miserable at work and to lose self-esteem. Bullying may take the form of intimidation, humiliation, public criticism or inconsistent expectations.[2] Doctors who are being bullied are reluctant to complain because they fear they may not get a good reference. Certainly, the historical record of whistle-blowers in the NHS provides no reassurance to anyone contemplating standing up to a bully.

Domestic problems such as divorce or financial difficulties can have an adverse effect on a doctor's work and are often combined with work-based issues to create stress. The doctor may have no outside interests or time to pursue any hobbies.

___ Clinical knowledge and skills

Some doctors are in trouble because of a lack of knowledge or a feeling that they are unable to apply their knowledge in a general practice setting. As Amery points out, the tools of general practice can become tyrants.[8] GPs can be motivated to improve performance by being given targets to achieve. However, if these become burdensome then the flow of the consultation is disturbed as the drive to record health prevention data prevents the GP from really listening to the patient. There has been an information explosion and with this has come a generation of expert patients. These patients have searched the net for information about their condition and have, as a result, high expectations of their GP's ability to solve their problem. Guidelines abound but they too can become tyrants and impair clinical judgement for the benefit of the individual patient. A writer of guidelines can have no concept of the specific context of the needs or best interests of the individual patient.[8] These developments can leave the doctor in a heightened state of anxiety about his or her lack of knowledge and the underlying threat of litigation.

General practitioners work in an environment of interruptions and clinical uncertainties. They may be placed in a situation where there is a conflict of interest between their financial interest in the practice and the clinical needs of the individual patient. For instance, a GP listening to the patient's story of her abusive husband may omit to record her blood pressure and smoking habits, thus affecting the practice income.

Working in clinical teams may be problematical when there is distrust, poor communication, unclear roles, unclear objectives, a lack of supervision and poor leadership. In this atmosphere a team can split, cliques are created and bullying can arise.

___ Factors affecting trainees' performance

Doctors entering their Foundation posts may feel unprepared for their new role by their medical undergraduate training.[9] Changes in working practices in the UK such as Modernising Medical Careers (MMC) and the European Working Time Directive (EWTD) have resulted in trainees having less clinical exposure and a fragmentation of traditional clinical teams and relationships. In such circumstances continuity of patient care has suffered. These changes have created new challenges for postgraduate medical education and mentoring.[10]

Personality traits that may help the trainee to cope with these challenges include: conscientiousness, extraversion, agreeableness, resilience and a deep learning style. Deep learning occurs when the trainee's imagination is captured and he or she pursues knowledge for its intrinsic interest, but this form of learning is not encouraged by high-stakes assessments. Other factors that affect the trainee's coping are his or her background experience: medical education, work experience, familiarity with language, culture and values. Their aptitude for their specialty is affected by abilities such as: pattern recognition, manual dexterity, tolerance of ambiguity, emotional intelligence and leadership.[10]

The stresses that trainees may experience can be summarised as:

- *personal pressures* – childcare responsibilities, working for postgraduate exams, family problems and financial difficulties can all affect the trainee's performance at work

- *health* – both mental and physical illness can affect how a trainee copes with his or her workload

- *context* – the workload and strictures of the EWTD have created extra pressure for young doctors

- *colleagues* – can be supportive but sadly sometimes there is bullying and harassment
- *patients' expectations* – patients can have high expectations and may complain when these are not met
- *training* – clinical pressures may leave little time for training.

___ Identifying a student or doctor in difficulty

Medical students and doctors who are struggling may have a history of problems with their knowledge, skills or attitude. Early identification and the provision of rapid support before a learner runs into difficulties is a goal of mentoring. One of the challenges is the fact that a student, trainee or doctor in difficulty may lack insight into his or her problem and so fail to seek help.

How to identify the struggling student

Students who are struggling may be identified by exam failure or poor performance during clinical attachments. Periods of absence or failure to respond to emails may also be signs of a struggling student; changes in behaviour or mood may also signal difficulties. The student may be frantically working excessive hours but be learning inefficiently. Under-performing students often do not seek support as they feel, mistakenly, that it is a sign of weakness. Consequently a mentor needs to see beyond a smiling face to detect hidden problems.[11]

Struggling students may have a poor attendance record, fail to submit work on time, or their clinical skills may not correspond to their stage of training. A student in difficulty may be achieving lower grades in assessments than predicted. They may not establish good relationships with patients or members of the healthcare team. They may be present at the back of a group and be unwilling to contribute to discussions. Their body language may reflect depression, anger or arrogance.

Students with mental health problems may exhibit any of the warning signs described. As in clinical practice, the mentor should be alert to any *change* of behaviour, for example a student who previously contributed to discussions who is now silent and withdrawn. Tearfulness, physical signs of self-harm, bizarre behaviour, high and low moods, and obvious excessive anxiety are all warning signs of possible underlying mental illness.

Early warning signs of a doctor in difficulty

Again, the mentor needs to look for evidence of change in the doctor's behaviour.[4] The doctor may disappear, arrive late or not answer bleeps or emails. There can be a fall off in clinical performance; they may be slow in clerking in patients or late in dictating letters. On occasions there may be angry outbursts on the ward, 'ward rage', which can be directed against colleagues, nurses or patients.[3] There may be corridor comments from colleagues about the doctor, which also can lead to a 'bypass syndrome' where team members avoid contacting the doctor for fear of his or her response. The doctor may become more rigid in his or her attitude and have little tolerance of uncertainty. The doctor may have problems with his or her career progress and feel disillusioned with medicine.

Concerns about a doctor may be raised during his or her appraisal or revalidation. Rarely, colleagues may raise concern with management about the doctor's behaviour. This problem is explored later in this chapter.[12,13]

___ How to respond to doctors in difficulty

A mentor should be empathic and take time to listen to the doctor's story.

Case story Mike

Mike is a GP registrar who performed well at medical school and following his Foundation years opts to train for general practice. He has no previous problems in his hospital jobs. He is keen to start surgeries on his own and explains to his educational supervisor that he has worked in Africa as a student and gained 'masses of experience'.

His educational supervisor is contacted by the practice nurse who is angry that Mike had told her that her asthma clinic was badly organised and that he could sort out a much better system for the patients. Several patients also spoke to other partners saying that the new doctor seemed very confident. He often changed their previous medication that they had been taking for years and had made disparaging comments about their previous care.

The educational supervisor feels a bit daunted in meeting Mike to tell him of these concerns because Mike is bright, has a tendency to arrogance, and never seems to admit to any faults. However, he arranges a meeting with Mike, setting aside an hour and requests that they should not be interrupted.

The educational supervisor begins by letting Mike know that he has come to the practice with excellent references from his previous posts and he wants to review his progress since working in a practice setting.

Mike agrees that he has enjoyed working both in hospital and general practice. When asked whether he felt there were any problems in his work, he says he has found some

51

of the patients were on treatment regimens that he felt were old fashioned, but that they seemed reluctant to take his advice to change their longstanding medication.

The educational supervisor remains silent.

Mike said, 'Oh yes, the practice nurse is seeing patients with asthma far too frequently and spending too much time chatting to them about their home situation, which I don't think is relevant.'

The supervisor asks how Mike had dealt with these issues. Mike explains that he just told patients that there were better treatments and that he had offered to organise a more efficient asthma clinic.

The supervisor said, 'Can I ask you a challenging question? How do you think that made the patients, their GPs and the nurse feel?'

Mike is quiet. 'I never gave that much thought. I suppose they would be grateful that I wanted to improve things for them.'

'Do you think they might have felt a bit undermined?' asked the supervisor. 'The patients might feel a lack of confidence in their treatment. Their GPs might be irritated that you had not consulted them before changing their treatment. The practice nurse might see your input as arrogant and interfering.'

Mike replied, 'No, I can see I might be a bit enthusiastic but never arrogant. Has anyone said I am arrogant?'

The educational supervisor replied, 'You are a bright young doctor who is enthusiastic and keen to make your mark in the practice. I think sometimes in your enthusiasm you fail to stop and think out the consequences of your actions on other people. General practice is a different setting from hospital and we all work as a close team. Perhaps you need to think a bit more about the other team members?'

'But have there been complaints about me? Will this affect my reference?'

'No, not complaints. A few patients were taken aback when you threw their previous medications into the bin. Belinda the practice nurse was a bit upset but she only told me so that I could give you some feedback. I want to suggest some helpful ways forward for you but would like to know whether you have any pressures or stresses at present either in the practice or in your home life.'

'I am relieved to hear what you say. I guess I can be a bit brash at times. There are no outside pressures. I am very happy at home with my wife who is expecting a baby in six months' time. I am grateful for your honest feedback. What do you suggest that I do in future?'

'I think perhaps just pausing a little more before plunging in with a suggestion. I think it might be helpful if you made a note of one or two situations where you felt you want to make changes and write down your feelings and the possible feelings of others involved. If you keep these reflections we can go over them in our next meeting.'

'Thank you. I will do that.'

The challenging trainee commonly has one or more of the following characteristics: lacking in insight, attitude problems, arrogance, communication problems, unrealistic expectations, bullying tendencies or mental health problems.[2] These doctors can monopolise the educational supervisor's and mentor's time. Intervening to provide support at an early stage will help both the trainee, his or her colleagues and patient care. If there has been a critical event that precipitates the problem the trainee should have feedback as soon as is practical. As described in Chapter 5, feedback should always include positive comments as well as addressing the negative issues. If conflict is anticipated then it is wise to have two people present, perhaps the educational supervisor and the mentor who can be an advocate and supporter of the trainee.

Additional communication strategies that can be helpful in enabling doctors to disclose their difficulties include:

- self-disclosing – by revealing difficulties you have faced, discussing past failures and your own vulnerabilities, you allow trainees to accept that all doctors face difficulties and carry burdens

- normalising – explaining that feeling uncertain is an integral part of general practice and can best be dealt with by an honest sharing of concerns

- reframing – discussing the problem allows the trainee to step out of him or herself and to see a problem from another person's perspective

- associating – drawing together different strands of the problem

- challenging – 'Can I ask you a strange question?'

- legitimising their concerns and giving permission to say things are difficult – 'How does this affect you?' 'What do you think might be going on?'

- exploring their Ideas, Concerns and Expectations (ICE)

- stressing that professional boundaries between a patient and doctor are explicit and clear.

Although parallels have been drawn between the mentor–mentee relationship and the doctor–patient relationship, there are specific differences. Students and trainees are not patients and, although the skills required to help may overlap, the relationship is different. The primacy of the patient in front of the doctor is central to patient care. The interests of a mentee, although important, do not come first. Patient care is a bigger priority.

___ Doctors in difficulty

Doctors in difficulty are too often just left to struggle because colleagues are reluctant to interfere, but this only builds more difficulties in the future. How much better it is to intervene earlier to help a colleague rather than to have to deal with a complex complaint at a later date.

General practice along with obstetrics and gynaecology and psychiatry are the specialties with most referrals to NCAS with doctors who are in difficulty. Male doctors over the age of 60 are most at risk of referral, while GPs over the age of 60 are seven times more likely to be referred than colleagues under 40 years of age. Doctors qualifying outside the UK are more at risk but this is not related to ethnicity but is related to their medical school of origin.[14]

___ Helping doctors in difficulty

In addition to mentoring there are a number of organisations that can be involved in helping a doctor in difficulty, such as the British Medical Association (BMA), NCAS and departments of occupational health. The doctor's own GP should be involved when the health of the doctor is in question. Mentoring is uniquely placed to help the doctor whose problem is not so serious as to necessitate referral to a regulating organisation or to an employer. A mentor, because he or she is not in a position to make a judgement about a doctor, can provide a confidential listening ear.

Box 4.1 Tips for helping doctors in difficulty[4]

- Don't ignore concerns.
- Be realistic.
- Follow process.
- Record everything.
- Don't let it get personal.

- Ask for help.
- Remain cheerful.
- Maintain confidentiality.
- Get help.

___ Raising concerns

However, if the problem of the doctor's behaviour or performance is serious or threatens patient safety the mentor needs to be aware of sources of help. *Good Medical Practice* states that doctors have a responsibility to act if they have genuine and significant concerns about the performance of a colleague.[15] Acting on concerns about colleagues is never easy, but may be necessary to protect patient safety, which is one of the primary responsibilities of healthcare professionals.

The following are examples of situations where a doctor should raise concerns:[16]

- poor management or administration that compromise patient safety
- lack of compliance with employment law and good human resource practice
- unacceptable behaviour (e.g. harassment or unlawful discrimination of staff or patients)
- situations that compromise compliance with professional codes of conduct for the individual or colleagues
- personal health problems of the practitioner leading to poor practice
- poor clinical performance
- ill treatment of a patient
- suspected fraud or suspected/actual criminal offence
- poor quality of care
- malpractice
- welfare of subjects in clinical trials
- acts of violence, discrimination or bullying towards patients
- acts of fraud
- doctors or other staff being mistreated by patients
- inappropriate relationships between patients and doctors
- illness that may affect a doctor's ability to practise in a safe manner
- substance and alcohol misuse affecting ability to work
- negligence
- fraud or corruption

- deliberate attempt to cover up any of the above.

Healthcare organisations are responsible for developing policies and procedures to recognise performance concerns early, and to act swiftly to address the concerns. Organisations sometimes appear to be reluctant to accept their responsibility for poorly performing doctors.[14, 17] Organisations that may be involved when there are serious concerns about a doctor's performance include:

- *deanery (Scotland), Health Education Team England,*
  the Postgraduate Medical Education and Training Board –
  these provide professional development programmes, coaching,
  career guidance and confidential counselling

- *occupational health* – for health issues including mental health,
  disability and dyslexia. It may recommend a period away from work,
  part-time working or changes to the working environment

- *General Medical Council* – regulation including fitness to practise,
  revalidation, misconduct, poor performance, criminal conviction,
  physical or mental health problems

- *NCAS* – addresses concerns of individual doctors and provides a
  support service for Trusts

- *defence organisations* – complaints, advice, ethical dilemmas,
  legal issues

- *BMA* – contract concerns, job plans, revalidation, stress.

Issues with training may be a cause for concern for both trainees and trainers, and postgraduate deaneries are empowered to address this type of concern. The postgraduate deanery and training programme director should be the first point of contact if speaking to the educational supervisor is unsuccessful. Each GP practice should have a clear policy on how to deal with concerns, including a named contact. Each Acute Trust should have a clear policy on how to consider concerns; the clinical director of the unit or the medical director may be approached in confidence.

___ Conclusion

Concerns about professional practice are more complex than at first sight.[13] It may be the reverse of 'What you see is what you get'; much of the problem is hidden and requires patience, kindness and empathy to elucidate. Many doctors are demoralised as a result of pressures and criticism from the public and media. Consideration must be given to providing more effective support for doctors. A requirement for every doctor to choose a mentor might be a positive first step. A good mentor has the ability to turn around a struggling student or doctor and change failure into success.[18]

Key points

The reasons underlying a doctor in difficulty are often complex.

Doctors need to pick up early signs of a colleague who is struggling.

A mentor is well placed to help doctors and students before serious problems arise.

Mentors should be approachable and non-judgemental.

Doctors have a duty to act if they have serious concerns about a colleague.

Resources

Useful web resources on raising concerns include the following:

- The BMA has whistleblowing guidance for doctors and medical students – http://bma.org.uk/practical-support-at-work/whistleblowing [accessed 25 June 2014]
- The BMA website also provides links to national and local sources of help for such conditions as illness, stress, distress, depression and addiction – http://bma.org.uk/practical-support-at-work/doctors-well-being/websites-for-doctors-in-difficulty [accessed 6 June 2014]
- Department of Health. *The Public Interest Disclosure Act 1998 (PIDA) – whistleblowing in the NHS*. Health Service Circular (HSC 1999/198). London: DH, 1999, www.gov.uk/government/publications/compromise-agreements-and-the-public-interest-disclosure-act-1998 [accessed 25 June 2014].

References

1 Knights J A, Kennedy B J. Medical school selection: screening for dysfunctional tendencies. *Medical Education* 2006; **40(11)**: 1058–64.

2 Cooper N, Forrest K. *Essential Guide to Educational Supervision in Postgraduate Medical Education*. London: BMJ Books, Wiley-Blackwell, 2009.

3 Chambers R, Wall D, Campbell I. Stress, coping mechanisms and job satisfaction in general practitioner registrars. *British Journal of General Practice* 1996; **46(407)**: 343–8.

4   McLaughlan C. *Managing Poor Performance and Doctors in Difficulty*. National Clinical Assessment Service, www.healthcareconferencesuk.co.uk/news/newsfiles/claire-mclaughlan-for-handbook_185.pdf   [accessed 25 June 2014].

5   Brooks S K, Chalder T, Gerada C. Doctors vulnerable to psychological distress and addiction: treatment from the Practitioner Health Programme. *Journal of Mental Health* 2011; **20(2)**: 157–64.

6   Firth-Cozens J. A perspective on stress and depression. In: J Cox, J King, A Hutchison, P McAvoy (eds), *Understanding Doctors' Performance*. Oxford: Radcliffe Publishing, 2006, pp. 22–37.

7   Alliott R. Facilitatory mentoring in general practice. *BMJ Careers Focus* 1996; **313**: S2–7060.

8   Amery J. *The Integrated Practitioner: turning tyrants into tools in health practice*. Oxford: Radcliffe Publishing, 2013.

9   Wall D, Bolshaw A, Carolan J. From undergraduate medical education to pre-registration house officer year: how prepared are students? *Medical Teacher* 2006; **28(5)**: 435–9.

10 Paice E. The role of education and training. In: J Cox, J King, A Hutchison, P McAvoy (eds), *Understanding Doctors' Performance*. Oxford: Radcliffe Publishing, 2006, pp. 78–90.

11 Dick J, Dixon R, Jeffrey D, McDonald L. *Getting Started … Struggling Students*. Dundee: Centre for Medical Education, University of Dundee, 2013.

12 Taylor C J, Houlston P, Wilkinson M. Mentoring for doctors in difficulty. *Education for Primary Care* 2012; **23(2)**: 87–9.

13 Paice E, Orton V. Early signs of the trainee in difficulty. *Hospital Medicine* 2004; **65(4)**: 238–40.

14 Old P, Scotland A. Doctors in difficulty. In: H Markar, G O'Sullivan (eds), *Medical Management: a practical guide*. London: Hodder Arnold, 2013, pp. 184–98.

15 General Medical Council. *Good Medical Practice*. London: GMC, 2013.

16 British Medical Association. Whistleblowing. http://bma.org.uk/practical-support-at-work/whistleblowing/raising-a-concern/when-do-i-act   [accessed 25 June 2014].

17 Miller A, Archer J. Impact of workplace assessments on doctors' education and performance: a systematic review. *British Medical Journal* 2010; **341**: 5064.

18 Lake J. Doctors in difficulty and revalidation: where next for the medical profession? *Medical Education* 2009; **43(7)**: 611–12.

FEEDBACK

5

"Just listen and the patient will tell you the diagnosis, if you give them enough time."

Dr W. Astley, a home visit in general practice

Most students and trainees feel that they do not receive sufficient feedback. Giving feedback is a core skill for a mentor and improves the mentee's performance.

Case story George

George is a newly appointed GP registrar. Following a surgery with his educational supervisor, Dr Brown, he meets Dr Brown at the end of surgery for feedback on his performance.

Dr Brown said, 'Thank you for asking for feedback, George. This must be quite different from working in your last post in elderly care medicine. How did you feel things went today?'

George replied, 'I wish I had diagnosed that child with chicken-pox. I felt such a twit!'

'We can chat about that in a little while. First tell me what you did really well.'

'Erm, well I listened to the woman with sleep problems and found she was quite depressed. I fixed up a longer appointment for her to come back and talk further in a couple of days.'

'Any other good points?'

'I was able to give that young teacher advice on the morning-after pill.'

'Yes, that consultation went well. You have a good listening manner and did not interrupt her. Also you examined the young child with the rash. Her mum had confidence in you because you spent a little time getting to know the child. Other good points I felt were that you were happy to look up and check drug doses, which is safe practice. You seemed quite relaxed about asking my opinion when you were puzzled by the chicken-pox rash. All this is very positive. Can we now look at things that might make your consultations even better?'

'Yes, that would be good. I want to learn.'

'Well, if you were doing the consultation again what might you do differently?'

'Well, I should have known that papular-vesicular rash was chicken-pox. I also felt a bit disappointed that I had to look up so many drug doses and get help with the prescriptions.'

'Good, those certainly were points to work on. Most doctors struggle with prescribing when coming into the general practice setting. You also took a long time working out the practice computer software. When two patients came in you were still looking at the screen inputting data from the previous consultation.'

'I did not realise. They must have thought I was very offhand. I will make sure that I familiarise myself with the computer software. I will also move that monitor screen on the desk so that there is no danger of seeming to ignore the patient.'

'Well done today, George, I am sure you are going to enjoy general practice. Let's agree a brief plan to review when I meet you in a fortnight. You are going to familiarise yourself with the practice software and pick up some prescribing tips. Would you like to sit in with me when I review some repeat prescriptions?'

'That was great. Thanks for your help. Yes, I would like help with the prescribing.'

It is through feedback that students and doctors are able to see themselves as others see them and so change their behaviour.[1] If feedback is to be effective there needs to be a climate of mutual respect. Establishing the ground rules is one way of creating such an environment (see Chapter 3). Mentors are not concerned with assessment, yet other tutors involved in giving feedback may also have an assessment role. It is important that feedback is not evaluative or judgemental otherwise the student or doctor receiving it may become defensive.

Feedback is concerned with improving clinical skills and providing reassurance about achieved competencies.[2] It should guide future learning and reinforce strengths as well as giving pointers for improvement. Feedback can also enhance professional development and encourage reflective practice. Students who do not receive feedback may assume that their practice is satisfactory. So feedback is not just vital for a doctor's learning but also for patient care.[2]

Feedback can take many forms. The following are sometimes described as Pendleton's Rules (see Table 5.1):[3]

Table 5.1 **Pendleton's Rules**

Prompt	Feedback should not contain surprises, so the closer to the event being discussed the better. However, if the situation being discussed has aroused strong emotions such as anger, it may be better to allow some time to pass for emotions to settle before giving sensitive feedback
Regular	Feedback should be a continuous process, so informal simple feedback should be given whenever the opportunity arises. Sadly, all too often tutors pick up on a student's or trainee's mistakes without making any positive comments
Sensitive	Mentors need first to ask the mentee what he or she felt went well. This gives the mentee self-confidence and the mentor an idea of the level of the person's self-awareness. The mentor should be specific and comment on observed behaviour without being judgemental. The mentor should never be aggressive and never be tempted to humiliate the individual. The student or trainee should identify at least one thing that he or she could improve on. This encourages the mentee to see that mistakes are an integral part of practice and that there is always room for improvement. The mentor then identifies at least one area for improvement. Once mentees have received affirmation of their skills they are happier to listen to constructive criticism that is aimed at helping their future performance
Honest	Feedback must be honest if it is to be helpful. Students and trainees want to know their weaknesses as well as their strengths
Followed up	Since the purpose of feedback is to improve performance the mentee and mentor should agree some specific goals that are measurable and agree a time for review

___ Giving difficult feedback

The general rules for giving feedback should still be followed when challenging unacceptable behaviour. Positive aspects should be discussed first. The mentor should be aware of any specific problems and other assessments of the mentee that have given rise to concern.

Case story **Craig**

Craig is a final-year medical student. He has been referred to the mentor, Martine, by the Medical School Administrator because the plagiarism software has picked up that his last case discussion was very similar to that of one of last year's students who is now a Foundation Year Doctor in the same unit where Craig is attached. When confronted by the administrator Craig flatly denies any plagiarism. Craig has not met

Martine before but he knows that the Administrator has informed the Teaching Dean of his concerns.

Before the meeting

Martine is aware that plagiarism is a serious issue that might result in a Fitness to Practise hearing. She downloads the university plagiarism policy to familiarise herself with the regulations before the meeting.

She looks up Craig's student record and finds that he has been an exemplary student, possibly in line for a distinction.

She speaks to the Administrator to see whether there is any doubt and how reliable the software is in detecting plagiarism. She gets a copy of Craig's essay and the other student's work with the areas of concern highlighted.

She also speaks to the Teaching Dean to get his view on the seriousness of the situation. He thinks a meeting with Martine might allow Craig the space to confide in the reason for the plagiarism.

Martine allows an hour for the meeting with Craig. After introductions she states the ground rules and explains that, if he wishes, the conversation can be entirely confidential. However, he might decide to allow her to discuss matters raised with the Teaching Dean, but only if he permits that to happen.

Craig looks pale and distraught, and is near to tears.

Martine began, 'Craig, it's good to meet you. I have seen your student record and know that you are a really good student. I know too that this is a horrible time for you. I have been asked to talk to you about the allegation of plagiarism.'

Craig replied, 'I know, it's crazy. Why would I copy anything?'

Martine said, 'Look, I am here on your side to help you. I have the relevant bits highlighted here. If you have not copied the other student's essay, you must not admit to anything you have not done. But if you have copied then it is much better that you own up and we can work out a way of dealing with the problem.'

Craig looks worried. 'But will I get my studies terminated? I could not face that.'

Craig begins to weep.

'No, it is highly unlikely that would happen with a first offence', said Martine. 'What would be more serious would be if you were dishonest about it because that becomes an issue of professional misconduct.'

Craig replied, 'OK, I have been a complete idiot. I knew the deadline for my case discussion was close. I have been very stressed because my father, who is an estate agent, is going bust. Things at home in Wales are really bad so I took a few days off to support my family. I just could not work. They were upset because they did not want anything to interfere with my studies. I did not know anyone I could talk to so when I came back I asked Bill (the FY1) if I could look at one of his last year's case discussions just to see what they were like. I was in such a rush that I did a cut and paste job on his case. I just panicked ... I know it was wrong and I am really sorry that I was so stupid. Is there anything I can do now?'

'Thank you for being honest with me. I am relieved that you have admitted your error and that you realise it is a serious mistake. It's much the best way to admit these things. I suggest that you rewrite the case discussion and resubmit it by next week. Is that a deadline you can manage?'

'Of course I will do that, but what about the plagiarism?'

'Well, I suggest you write a page reflection on your plagiarism and what you have learned from this experience. I am happy to look at it and then you could send that in to the Teaching Dean with a letter of apology, including the extenuating circumstances and a commitment never to do this again. I will speak to the Teaching Dean, if that's OK with you, and recommend that this goes no further and that you are sorry and have learned from this experience. I will get back to you by email to arrange another meeting to make sure that things have been resolved.'

'Thank you. I would be pleased if you would speak to the Teaching Dean. I will get the letter to him done today. I would be grateful if you would look at my reflective writing. I find it difficult.'

After the meeting: The mentor makes a detailed record of what had been said and the agreed action plan. She spoke to the Teaching Dean and explains she had Craig's consent to tell him what has happened, explains the extenuating circumstances and describes his genuine remorse.

Follow-up meeting

The Teaching Dean agrees not to take things any further and the matter is now closed. It will not affect Craig's final assessment.

These are examples of formal feedback. Feedback may also take place on an informal basis as part of everyday clinical practice. A trainee doctor performing a clinical procedure such as catheterisation may get immediate feedback from the registrar with a comment on things that went well and a practical tip on how make it even better next time.

____ Potential barriers to effective feedback

- Feedback can come as a shock when the mentee and learner do not share the same objectives or when it is given in an unstructured way.

- If feedback is limited to negative judgements that the mentee perceives as being unfair.

- If the mentee has had bad experiences of feedback in the past and sees the meeting as an opportunity to defend his or her position.

- If insufficient time has been set aside for the feedback.

___ 360° degree feedback

All feedback gives students or doctors an opportunity to see themselves as others see them. While individual one-to-one feedback is the gold standard, 360° feedback involves colleagues, other doctors, nurses, other healthcare professionals and administrative staff giving their feedback to the trainee. This gives doctors new knowledge of their contribution to the team and how other team members see doctors interacting with them.

___ Conclusion

This chapter has highlighted the importance of giving feedback in a proper way to ensure it is effective in promoting learning, developing professionalism and encouraging reflection.[4] The next chapter looks at another core skill for a mentor, to encourage reflective practice.

Key points

Students value feedback.

Giving constructive feedback is a core skill for a mentor.

Always start with positive feedback.

Feedback gives students and doctors insight into how others see them.

___ References

1   Hicks R, McCracken J. How to give difficult feedback. *Physician Executive* 2011; **37(3)**: 84–7.

2   Gigante J, Dell M, Sharkey A. Getting beyond 'Good job': how to give effective feedback. *Pediatrics* 2011; **127(2)**: 205–7.

3   Pendleton D, Schofield T, Tate P, Havelock P. *The Consultation: an approach to learning and teaching.* Oxford: Oxford University Press, 1984.

4   Donnelly P, Kirk P. How to ... give effective feedback. *Education for Primary Care* 2010; **21(4)**: 267–9.

6

REFLECTION

"I wish doctors would relax and write what they feel."
Bobbie Farsides, philosopher, marking a masters assignment

___ Reflection

The mentor can facilitate learning by encouraging the mentee (student, trainee or general practitioner) to reflect on his or her practice. For the beginner 'doing reflection' may seem a bit of a mechanical exercise, moving round the reflective cycle: experience, reflect, plan, change, implement and begin the cycle all over again. Initially reflection is *on* an action or experience but then develops into reflection *in* action, while in the situation.[1] Reflection may be taken further to increase self-awareness or become mindful. Mindfulness encompasses an ability to see the bigger picture. This form of practical wisdom opens new possibilities for learning. Reflection can be a tool for reconnecting with caring ideals and an understanding of one's emotions.

There are many definitions of reflection. Most include ideas of the ability of doctors to think critically about their own reasoning decisions, enquiry and translation skills.[2] The General Medical Council highlights the need for doctors to be reflective.[3] Reflection is about personal and professional growth by thinking about one's practice in a structured way.

A mentor needs to be aware of models of reflection. Gibbs describes a cycle of reflection (see Figure 6.1).[4]

Case story **Kirsty**
....

Kirsty is a final-year student who regards reflection as a tick-box exercise. She comes to her mentor for advice on writing a reflection for her finals portfolio. The mentor uses the Gibbs cycle as a framework for her reflection.

Figure 6.1 **Gibbs reflective cycle**

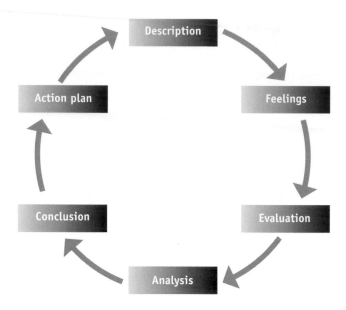

Description

Kirsty writes describing a clinical incident that made her feel uncomfortable. 'It was in a busy out-patient clinic. The consultant told this young woman that her breast cancer had recurred and that she would need further chemotherapy. The consultant then said she was going out to get the specialist nurse to talk to her and answer her questions. I was left with the patient who broke down as soon as the consultant left the room. I felt so distressed for her. She had a young family. I found my own eyes filling up and I did not know what to say. It was so awful for both of us.'

Feelings

The mentor acknowledges the difficulty of the situation and asked Kirsty, 'You say it was awful. Can you tell me a bit more about your feelings?'

Kirsty said, 'I felt so embarrassed and distressed. This poor woman had been given terrible news and was just left with me. I had never seen her before and knew very little about her other than she had young children. I felt inadequate. I did not know what to say. I was angry at the consultant. Why had she just left the room?'

Evaluation

The mentor asks Kirsty what was good or bad about this experience.

'Well, I suppose it was good that the consultant trusted me enough to allow me to sit in on the consultation where she was breaking bad news', replied Kirsty. 'What was bad was that I was disappointed that I got so emotionally involved and personally distressed. It was bad that I was not able to comfort the patient but just sat there looking very sad. I feel so guilty.'

Analysis

The mentor asks Kirsty to think about what sense she can make of her reactions.

Kirsty reflects. 'Talking about this with you today I can see that I got really distressed because I over-identified with the patient. Instead of being able to help her I was overwhelmed with the news. I kept thinking, "What would that be like for me?" I am a bit sensitive about this as my auntie died three years ago with breast cancer and this patient's bad news brought all that back too. One good thing I suppose was that I did not leave the room with the consultant. The patient may have received some comfort from my presence.'

Conclusion

The mentor picks up on this last comment and emphasises how well Kirsty did to stay with the patient. Many doctors cope with distressing situations by distancing themselves from patients. This is unhelpful for both patient and doctor. The mentor also comments that doctors often have guilty feelings, mostly because they care so much and consequently set such high standards for themselves.

The mentor asked Kirsty, 'What else could you have done?'

'Thinking about that, what I should have done was to imagine what it was like for the patient, with her situation, not what it would have been like for me. I think it is good to share the patient's emotion but at the same time I have to remember the patient is not me, nor my auntie. If I get too overwhelmed with my own distress I am not able to help her.'

Action plan

The mentor emphasised how important it is that Kirsty retains her empathic skills of sharing emotions with the patient and trying to see things from the patient's perspective. At the same time there is a balance to achieve in recognising that the patient and self are different and that it is important to keep this perspective in mind. She asks Kirsty what she would do in a similar situation in future.

Kirsty replied, 'I will ask the patient if she wants anyone to be with her when I break bad news. I would stay with the patient after breaking the news to support her and make sure she had access to support afterwards. I am not so worried about showing emotion after my chat with you today. I can see the difference in taking the patient's perspective and being personally distressed. When I am a Foundation Doctor, I will try not to leave a student in the same situation, and I will check that he is feeling OK about being invited into a bad news consultation. I can see how helpful it is to have someone to talk to and I will make sure I too can find someone to talk to about distressing situations.'

The mentor then reflected. 'We are engaging in reflective practice. Although talking about it is valuable for both of us, it is even better if you keep a written record of some of the salient points in this story. I would suggest particularly that you record your feelings.'

'Yes, I will do that. I have learned a lot today, not just about the case but about the value of reflection.'

Guided reflection allows the mentee to receive feedback and to evolve a plan for future action. The reflection is not simply a cycle but more like a spiral because there will be a chance to come back after the student encounters a similar situation. She can consider whether the new actions have worked better and learn from that. With practice these steps become less laboured and more automatic.

There are many other models of reflection. Johns recommends guided reflection, suggesting the following areas for questions.[1]

Johns model for structured reflection

- What information do I need to access to learn through this experience?

- What was the experience? A description emphasising the context and clarifying key issues.

- What am I trying to achieve? Why? What are the consequences? What are the feelings generated, in the patient and in me?

- What other influencing factors are relevant? Internal or external?

- Did I have enough knowledge?

- Could I have dealt better with the situation?

- What choices did I have?

- How will I move on next time?

Although reflection is often triggered by negative experiences it is often helpful to look at a clinical problem that was dealt with well.

___ The reflective practitioner

Johns asks, 'What does it mean to be a reflective practitioner?' It involves moving from a beginner who 'does' reflection by thinking about an action, almost as a tick-box exercise, to an ability to reflect in action, a form of 'thinking on one's feet'. Then one can progress to a form of mindful practice, in which the reflective practitioner's practical wisdom encompasses a broader perspective of the situation.[1] Reflection evolves by learning through experience to gain new insights and practical wisdom. The reflective practitioner has clinical curiosity and is open to new possibilities. Every clinical experience is an opportunity for new learning and reflection. With its emphasis on expressing and understanding feelings, reflection provides a good route to reconnecting with caring ideals.

___ The transition from novice to expert

In the journey from novice to expert there are many transition points. The novice becomes the advanced beginner who, in turn, becomes competent, progressing to proficiency and finally with much experience to expertise. One of the goals of education is to inspire lifelong reflective learning. Reflection and feedback facilitate learning but many students and trainees feel that they do not receive sufficient experience of such training. For instance, a mistaken assumption is often made that they understand the concept of reflection.[2]

It is disconcerting to discover that many senior medical students have low levels of self-esteem. The mentoring relationship provides a context in which to build students' and trainees' self-confidence and demonstrate the use of guided reflection. Where reflection becomes too institutionalised it may become a burdensome exercise and lose all value as a learning tool. Indeed, excessive self-reflection may reduce insight if it becomes purely a rumination on problems.

Johns characterises the novice learner as exhibiting linear thinking in action, viewing the parts of his or her experience in isolation. Novices rely on an external authority who has the 'right' answer. They see themselves as distinct from the situation they face and they are uncomfortable with uncertainty.[1] In contrast, reflective practitioners are intuitive in their practice, adopting a holistic approach and do not need to rely on some external authority. The reflective practitioner is always learning from experience, seeing him or herself as an integral part of the clinical situation.[5] He or she tolerates uncertainty and sees 'not knowing' as a part of practical wisdom. A mentor can help the student or trainee to shift from a position of seeing reflection as a tiresome cognitive activity with little benefit, to a more meditative activity that is achieved through quiet contemplation.[1]

___ Some problems facing reflection in practice

People need time to reflect on their practice. Mentees need a chance to look at their practice not just in functional terms of what we do but also to look at the philosophical aspects of how their values correspond with their practice. Schön's vision of the reflective practitioner includes both technical competency and artistic expression.[5] Notions of critical reflection also include being wise, which includes the ability to cope with uncertain knowledge and understand the fallibility of knowledge. Wisdom is also associated with good clinical judgement, a depth of knowledge and experience.

There is a danger that reflection may be reduced simply to a matter of professionalism rather than a dynamic activity that enhances learning and caring. This trend may in part be due to the influence of a Western culture emphasising analysis and problem solving. An Eastern view would be to adopt an approach of integration and contemplation. Reflective practitioners put their relationship with a mentee or a patient at the centre of their practice and attempt to negotiate shared meanings.

Amery asks, 'Have reflective tools become unbalanced and tyrannical?'[6] He suggests there may be a risk in asking experts consciously to reduce and analyse the systems and processes they are subconsciously using. Perhaps there is a pressure on them to regress from the automated, effortless and subconscious thinking of experts to the deliberate, effortful and conscious level of beginners.[6] As we become more expert, knowledge we had to keep at the front of our conscious mind (explicit knowledge) gradually slips to the unconscious mind (implicit knowledge).[7] As we acquire more experience, tasks that once required deliberative approaches gradually become routinised. Knowledge becomes tacit rather than explicit. Practice becomes a dance between the tacit and the explicit to check that the implicit practice is safe.[6] Experts are not defined by just what they know but how they apply what they know.

Eraut suggests that, as a doctor becomes more expert, the way he or she practises progresses from a conscious, deliberative process to one that is rapid and intuitive. Finally, this can develop into an instant and reflex response. Awareness also becomes more sophisticated, progressing from a need for conscious reflective monitoring to implicit monitoring and short, reactive reflection.[7] Amery suggests that it is not a question of the doctor ceasing to reflect but rather reflection itself that becomes subconscious and effortless once he or she becomes an experienced practitioner. Indeed, in that situation if experts try too hard to reflect they may risk paralysing their practice.[6]

___ Learning styles

Mentors should be aware of the principles of adult learning. Learners are self-directed and capable of determining their own educational needs. Their experience is a rich resource for learning. They value learning that is closely related to their own personal goals and which can be applied to their practice. A mentor needs to understand the range of factors influencing effective learning.

Mentees will have different learning styles. Some will be deep learners who embrace new ideas and look for meaning and concepts to link these to their existing knowledge. Others may be surface learners who accept facts uncritically and try to memorise them using rigid formulas. Strategic learners on the other hand tend to work to pass assessments rather than gaining a deeper understanding.

___ Narrative reflection

Narrative reflection is a means of increasing self-awareness by written reflection on the mentee's or patient's stories. This form of writing can help to make sense of the lives of patients, families, colleagues and oneself. Charon writes:

> *Patients want doctors who comprehend what they go through and who as a result stay the course with them through their illness. A medical practitioner without genuine awareness of what their patients go through may fulfil its technical goals but it is an empty medicine.*[8]

The emotional content of the learning process can also be explored within a mentoring relationship. Mentees need time and encouragement to ask questions such as 'How do I feel about this issue?' or 'Why do I feel this way?' With appropriate guidance they can develop their ability to understand their own feelings and those of others.

Written reflection can increase the mentee's self-awareness of his or her practice. Using the qualitative research paradigm, narrative reflection tries to make sense of what he or she experiences by paying attention to the meanings people give to their social encounters.[9] In a clinical sense it is making sense of the lives and experiences of patients, families, colleagues and other healthcare professionals. Making sense requires interpretation and is subjective. Explicitly analysing stories is a way of understanding both the self and others involved in the story.[10]

Narrative has the capacity to mobilise our consciousness and feelings, and helps to identify what it is to be human. It can result in a moral awakening that allows a chance to reassess the meanings of both the mentor's and mentee's experiences. Narrative reflection enables trainees to reconsider the professional and personal challenges that they have met in practice. If the reflection is discussed with the mentor it can be a powerful way of reframing the experience to provide valuable lessons for future practice.

For example, in clinical medicine, 'History writing' admits none of the doctor's feelings. The medical notes communicate meaning in a technologically efficient manner. There is no room for communicating what it is like to empathise with a patient or his or her family, no place to record the rage that was felt after the death of a patient that moved the doctor. Charon suggests 'Parallel notes' in the patient's record where there is an opportunity for doctors to write about emotions.[8]

Narrative reflection gives trainees permission to write about their experiences, thoughts, feelings, values and concerns, and enables them to create a meaningful process of engagement with their clinical world. Giving this permission to be 'human' and connected to a patient is central to reflective writing.[9]

___ Reflection and culture

The health agenda is now dominated by a management culture of consumerism that appears to value productivity above caring. Indeed, 'caring' activity can be perceived to be the responsibility of unqualified staff. This ignores the basic fact that suffering is caused by a lack of caring. In recent years in the NHS there have been a number of high-profile incidents showing a deplorable lack of care.[11] There is a need for a paradigm shift in the cultural values of NHS management to value holistic caring, creativity and collaborative teamwork. Guided reflection challenges the *status quo* of cold professional detachment. It allows healthcare professionals to voice their feelings and to empathise with their patients, resulting in better health for both.

Key points

Mentors can facilitate reflective learning.

Reflection should not be a burden.

Narrative reflection can help doctors to express their feelings.

Reflection is needed in the transition from novice to expert.

____ **References**

1   Johns C. *Becoming a Reflective Practitioner.* Oxford: Wiley-Blackwell, 2004.

2   Muir F. The understanding and experience of students, tutors and educators regarding reflection in medical education: a qualitative study. *International Journal of Medical Education* 2010; **1**: 61–7.

3   General Medical Council. *Tomorrow's Doctors.* London: GMC, 2009.

4   Gibbs G. *Learning by Doing: a guide to teaching and learning methods.* Oxford: Further Education Unit, 1988.

5   Schön D. *Educating the Reflective Practitioner.* San Francisco: Jossey-Bass, 1987.

6   Amery J. *The Integrated Practitioner: food for thought.* Oxford: Radcliffe Publishing, 2014.

7   Eraut M. Non-formal learning and tacit knowledge in professional work. *British Journal of Educational Psychology* 2000; **70(1)**: 113–36.

8   Charon R. *Narrative Medicine: honoring the stories of illness.* Oxford: Oxford University Press, 2006.

9   Feest K. Introducing narrative reflection. In: N Cooper, K Forrest (eds), *Essential Guide to Educational Supervision in Postgraduate Medical Education.* London: BMJ Books, Wiley-Blackwell, 2009, pp. 95–106.

10 Lincoln Y. Emerging criteria for quality in qualitative and interpretive research. *Qualitative Inquiry* 1995; **1(3)**: 275–89.

11 Francis R. *Report of the Mid Staffordshire NHS Foundation Trust Public Inquiry.* London: Stationery Office, 2013, www.midstaffspublicinquiry.com [accessed 25 June 2014].

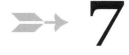

ROLE MODEL 7

"Sounds as though the palliative care team should be involved."
Dr Sean Elyan, during the oncology multidisciplinary ward meeting

___ Introduction

Role models are people with whom we identify and who have qualities we would like to share.[1] They can fashion the attitudes and behaviour of students and young doctors. They are, therefore, a fundamental part of developing professionalism. Excellence in role modelling demands high standards of clinical competency, teaching and empathy.

Students and young doctors identify with enthusiasm and compassion. They also admire openness, integrity and good relationships with patients in role models.[1] However, role models may not all be positive. Unfortunately, some senior doctors show poor attitudes or unethical behaviour, which distresses young doctors.[1] These issues are considered further in Chapter 11.

Role models can be distinguished from mentors because they teach by example whereas mentors have a formal relationship with mentees.[2] Although mentors may be role models, their role in developing professionalism is broader. Mentors actively engage in an explicit relationship with their junior colleagues, a relationship that evolves over time.[1]

Role modelling takes place in the formal, informal and hidden curriculum.[3] The hidden curriculum is a set of influences that functions at the level of organisational culture and includes the customs, rituals and taken-for-granted aspects of medicine that are unarticulated and unexplored.[4]

Lempp describes some possible unfortunate consequences of the hidden curriculum that may occur from negative role modelling:[4]

- loss of idealism

- adoption of a ritualised professional identity

- blocking of emotions, distancing

75

- acceptance of hierarchy.

  In Lempp's study of students' views of their teaching, four themes emerged. The first theme was:

- positive role models who offer encouragement.

  Themes of negative role models also emerged:

- haphazard teaching

- standing on hierarchy, e.g. teaching by humiliation

- encouraging competition rather than collaboration.

  Good role models have an integral part to play in correcting the last three themes above. Students should be welcomed and teachers prepared to teach. Humiliation is never an acceptable way to treat a student or doctor.

  Do students and young doctors emulate their role models? Sinclair's research suggests that students learned an aversion to exploring the patient's social and psychological problems in the course of their training.[5] He found that the students' personal idealism waned as they became absorbed in the culture of the profession and distanced from their family and non-medical friends. Sinclair also found that the students lacked self-awareness of the internal stress that must be associated with these changes. He found there was a gulf between the standards to which the students professed they sought and the qualities that they emulated.[5] It might be that a reliance on role models to teach students professionalism simply creates a culture that is resistant to change, but a change in culture is needed to make doctors aware of the patient's agenda. Whenever a medical intervention is considered, the student or doctor should ask him or herself, 'Does this intervention fit in with the patient's goals?'

  Wright found that students and young doctors valued the following qualities in a role model: integrity, a positive attitude to junior colleagues and compassion for patients.[6] They also identified the following as positive attributes: clinical competency, enthusiasm for their subject and teaching ability. It is interesting that research achievement and academic status were not considered as important. Those doctors who were rated highly as role models were ones who spent more time teaching and conducting ward rounds, and who stressed the importance of the doctor–patient relationship. They also found that clinicians who were thought of highly as role models were ones who were willing to share their professional experiences and their personal feelings.[1,6] A survey of GPs found that a positive attitude to teaching and an excellent doctor–patient relationship were considered important aspects of good role models.[7] Another study divided the attributes of a role model into three parts: physician, teacher and person. Attributes of the physician included enthusiasm, clinical reasoning and a good doctor–patient relationship. The teacher's valued characteristics were enthusiasm, involving the students and good communication. Personal values were enthusiasm, compassion and competence. Again, power, status and high earning ability did not feature as desirable characteristics of a good role model.[8]

Case story Matthew

Matthew, a consultant surgeon, is a mentor and role model for Foundation Doctors and students. He is approachable and has a sense of humour. He takes an interest in students and makes them feel welcome on his ward. He spends time ensuring that new doctors to the team have an induction. His surgical skills are exemplary and he never seeks to promote himself. Indeed he has disclosed that he had difficulties as a student, almost failing his second-year exam in anatomy.

He uses every opportunity to teach, including clerking patients himself and comparing notes with the Foundation Doctor. He never humiliates students or doctors if they display a lack of knowledge, supporting his team in the decisions they take. This gives them great confidence and helps to reduce stress. He just regards this role as a learning opportunity not only for the students but also for himself. His communication skills with patients are excellent and he allocates time to speak to relatives.

He is interested in his students' aspirations for the future and helps them to network with colleagues so that they can obtain good experience on electives. He takes time out with the doctors on his team to eat together in the hospital canteen or to have a coffee together in the hospital café.

By his professionalism, humility, his regard for patients and his respect for colleagues Matthew is a good example of an excellent role model. Many of those who worked with this surgeon kept in touch with him throughout their professional careers.

Attributes of a positive role model can be summarised as follows.

- An excellent level of clinical knowledge and skills with a patient-centred approach that models empathic behaviour.

- Teaching skills, in particular establishing rapport with learners, and being committed to their development. The teaching occurs in a supportive learning environment.

- Personal qualities include a positive 'can do' approach, integrity and an ability to inspire learners. Positive role models tend to be more conscientious, better team workers and able to cope with stressful situations.[9]

___ Career advice

Mentors can influence students' career choices even though they may not intentionally try to recruit students to join their specialties; students seem to be influenced by the role model's love of his or her work.[8] Mentors need to give mentees the opportunity to discuss their career choices. Too often this is left until the student or doctor has a problem with the career path he or she has chosen. Career advice should be an integral part of medical training. The mentor can also help the mentee network with doctors in their chosen specialty to gain experience.

Career advice services exist at university and in the deaneries. In Chapter 1 the Career Development Unit at Oxford was described as an example of innovation in this area.[10] The educational supervisor and College advisers may also offer career advice. Part of this advisory role might involve looking at the mentee's CV and helping with a practice interview. It is surprising how often students and young doctors do not do themselves justice in an interview simply because they have had no practice and have no idea what to expect.

Case story Melanie

Melanie is a final-year student from Hong Kong. She asks her mentor for a short practice viva before her finals. The finals viva is based on her portfolio of experience during her final two years at medical school. This is a high-stakes exam.

The mentor asks to see Melanie's portfolio even though it is incomplete. She books a room for half an hour and tells Melanie she will have a 20 minute viva and ten minute feedback. Both Melanie and Maxine the mentor dress for a finals exam to make the situation as realistic as possible.

After keeping Melanie waiting for five minutes Maxine calls her to the viva.

'Good afternoon Melanie', said Maxine. 'Thank you for your portfolio, which is an excellent piece of work. Can you tell me something you are really proud of or have enjoyed in your training?'

Melanie looks stunned. 'Erm well I enjoy everything. It's difficult to pick one thing.'

'OK, well I read your case report on diabetic ketoacidosis. Can you just tell me what happens physiologically in this condition?'

Melanie looks alarmed and bursts into tears. 'My mind has just gone blank ... I know the biochemical changes in DKA but I can't think straight.'

Maxine replied, 'Melanie, you were clearly thrown by my first question so let's take a few minutes to reflect on this part of the interview and then we can restart.'

'Oh I was awful! But you are right. I did not expect that first question and I find it very difficult to talk about things I have done well. I just feel under so much pressure. My parents have booked the flight and hotel to come to my graduation as they just seem to think it's bound to happen.'

'Well Melanie, reading your portfolio I think they are right but let us go through the viva a bit more. The examiners will try to put you at ease so you need to have a case that you are happy to talk about. I would advise not choosing your elective in Hong Kong but something in the course here. You also need to think about something that did not go well and be prepared to talk about it and say what you have learned. Think about areas for future learning as a Foundation Doctor. Remember that the examiners want you to pass. They are examining the quality of their teaching too. It's not just about you. Remember to look up and smile. You are a good student, so be proud of your work and show them how good you really are.'

'Thanks so much. I feel such a fool ... still it's better this happened today and not in the real viva.'

'Exactly – that's why we practise. Lots of students dry up or cry in these practices, so please don't feel bad about that. Shall we give it another go? Now Melanie, tell me something really good in your portfolio.'

'I enjoyed working on the ethics case of the patient I met with advanced pancreatic cancer. She asked me if there were any doctors here who would help her to die.'

'How did you react?'

'Well, I was taken aback. I am only a student. But she just wanted to talk. I just made sure she had as much privacy as possible and sat beside her and listened to her distress. She was not in pain but felt she was a burden to her family. She asked me about my family and I told her about my grandparents in Hong Kong who were very frail but we all loved them very much and it was a privilege to be able to look after them. We did not think of them as a burden ever.'

'What happened then?'

'The patient smiled and said that was a kind thing to say and it made her feel much better. I told her the staff admired the way she coped with her illness and she should feel free to tell us if she is in any pain or if she wants to talk about what might happen. The patient said that would be good, no she was not in pain but she would like to ask her consultant what she thought was likely to happen. I asked her if there was anything else I could help with today and the lady said no but thank you for listening to me.'

'Thank you, Melanie. I enjoyed reading your debate about assisted suicide. Now, is there anything in your portfolio which you are not so happy with which show that you need further training?'

'I will need to perform some of my practical procedures. I am not completely confident taking arterial blood gases and sometimes have difficulty with urinary catheterisation.'

'How will you address these issues?' asked Maxine.

'I will speak to my educational supervisor', replied Melanie, 'and ask the registrar if there are any opportunities to carry out these procedures on the ward. I will ask the registrar or FY2 to observe me and to provide feedback on my performance.'

At the conclusion of the practice viva Maxine gives Melanie some feedback on her performance and adds a few tips on coping with vivas. She offers a further meeting if Melanie feels she needs more help.

Melanie passed her final exams.

___ Conclusion

Excellent role models will always inspire students and doctors to develop professionally, particularly in areas of the informal and the hidden curriculum. As Paice *et al.* ask, 'Will these attitudes and behaviours prepare them for the health service of today?'[1]

A result of the Francis Inquiry has been to highlight the need for doctors and other healthcare professionals to see the world from the patient's view: a need for more empathy.[11] Role models will therefore need to demonstrate excellent team working skills and be willing to examine their own professionalism in the light of changing patient expectation. Doctors need to be more open to admit their vulnerabilities, to learn from nurses and other healthcare professionals, and to listen to patients.[1] Changing the current culture of the medical profession will not be easy but mentors could play a vital role in giving students and doctors the time and space to reflect on their attitudes and behaviours. All doctors should be part of a mentoring relationship and have the opportunity to reflect on their performance and how it can be improved.[1]

Key points

Role models can influence the attitudes and behaviour of students and doctors.

Negative role models cause students and doctors distress.

Positive role models show enthusiasm, compassion and competency.

Role models should demonstrate good interdisciplinary teamwork.

Mentors and role models could facilitate a change in the paternalistic NHS culture.

—— References

1   Paice E, Heard S, Moss F. How important are role models in making good doctors? *British Medical Journal* 2002; **325(7366)**: 707–10.

2   Ricer R E. Defining preceptor, mentor, and role model. *Family Medicine* 1998; **30(5)**: 328.

3   Hafferty FW. Beyond curriculum reform: confronting medicine's hidden curriculum. *Academic Medicine* 1998; **73(4)**: 403–7.

4   Lempp H, Seale C. The hidden curriculum in undergraduate medical education: qualitative study of medical students' perception of teaching. *British Medical Journal* 2004; **329(7469)**: 770–3.

5   Sinclair S. *Making Doctors: an institutional apprenticeship.* Oxford: Berg, 1997.

6   Wright S. Examining what residents look for in their role models. *Academic Medicine* 1996; **71(3)**: 290–2.

7   Lublin J R. Role modelling: a case study in general practice. *Medical Education* 1992; **26(2)**: 116–22.

8   Ambrozy D M, Irby D M, Bowen J L, *et al.* Role models' perceptions of themselves and their influence on students' specialty choices. *Academic Medicine* 1997; **72(12)**: 1119–21.

9   Passi V, Johnson S, Reile E, *et al.* Doctor role modelling in medical education: BEME guide no. 27. *Medical Teacher* 2013; **35(9)**: 1422–36.

10 Career Development Unit (CDU). www.oxforddeanerycdu.org.uk/about/about_cdu.html   [accessed 25 June 2014].

11 Francis R. *Report of the Mid Staffordshire NHS Foundation Trust Public Inquiry.* London: Stationery Office, 2013, www.midstaffspublicinquiry.com [accessed 25 June 2014].

FACING FAILURE: EXAMS AND ASSESSMENT 8

"Try general practice, but I think you will come back to paediatrics."
Dr James Syme, paediatrician

___ Introduction

Helping students and doctors with academic difficulties is a core part of the mentoring relationship. A failed exam is a common reason for a student or trainee to seek the help of a mentor or to be referred for such help.[1] A recent report on the mental health of students observes, 'early adult life is a crucial stage in the transition from adolescence to independence as an adult. Underachievement or failure at this stage can have long term effects on self-esteem and the progress of a person's life.'[2]

A mentor needs to have an understanding of the student's approach to study and learning style. Universities encourage a deep learning that is motivated by a desire to understand and to see the relevance of learning. This type of learning is revealed as the student reflects on his or her experience and integrates material from different disciplines. In contrast, surface learning is superficial, motivated by a fear of failure and consists of a regurgitation of facts. Paradoxically, a surface learning style is predictive of failure.[3] Strategic learning is motivated by a desire for success and characterised by competition with others.

Medical education aims not simply for competency but also for capability. Competency is concerned with what an individual is able to do in terms of knowledge, skills and attitudes. Capability is a broader concept, which is a measure of the extent to which an individual can adapt to change, generate new knowledge and continue to improve his or her performance.[4] Mentoring is a powerful way of enhancing capability through feedback, and teaching that accepting failure is part of progress.

It provides a balance between support and appropriate challenge. Learning that builds capability develops when individuals engage with uncertainty and new information. A transformation occurs in which existing competencies are adapted and tested in new circumstances; capability is developed with experience, mentoring, feedback and reflection.[4] Deep learners are receptive to feedback and can adapt appropriately to change. Superficial learners may reject feedback and reflection, and consequently do not adapt their behaviour appropriately. The capable doctor is a person who can access information effectively, linking seemingly unrelated areas and has a holistic approach to the patient. These doctors can make sense of a problem by using intuition and imagination, acknowledging complexity. This type of problem solving is a creative process that can be enhanced through effective mentoring. This form of creative approach requires trust between the mentor and mentee, which can be facilitated by setting and agreeing ground rules from the outset (Chapter 3).

Case story Sarah

Sarah, a third-year student, finds online EMI multiple-choice exams very difficult. She passed her clinical exams comfortably but only achieves low marks in multiple-choice online tests.

A sample question

Theme: **Neurosurgery**

Options:

A. Chronic subdural haemorrhage	**F.** Meningioma
B. Secondary brain tumour	**G.** Subarachnoid haemorrhage
C. Astrocytoma	**H.** Acute subdural haemorrhage
D. Extradural haemorrhage	**I.** Pituitary adenoma
E. Oligodendroglioma	**J.** Intracerebral haemorrhage

Lead in: select the most likely diagnosis
Questions

1   A previously well 79-year-old woman is brought into hospital after her husband noticed she had become increasingly confused and drowsy over the past week. Her husband says she slipped on ice several weeks ago but doesn't recall any falls in the past week.

   Answer = A

2   A 26-year-old man presents to his GP after noticing his vision has reduced laterally. Upon questioning he has been experiencing headaches for the past month and has recently noticed a milk-like fluid leaking from his nipples.

Answer = I

3   A 23-year-old woman has been involved in a low-velocity car accident. She appears well when paramedics arrive but despite this they decide to take her to A&E for a more full assessment. After initially being very chatty she suddenly loses consciousness in the ambulance and her GCS drops from 15 to 9.

Answer = D

The mentor watches as Sarah talks through how she approached the paper.

Sarah said, 'I look at the answers, then panic a bit, then look at the questions and try to answer them.'

'What do you do when you finish?' replied the mentor.

'Oh I go through and find that I have got loads wrong and change my answers.'

'What about trying a new approach? I would like you to read the next question but cover up the answers. The stem might ask for the most likely diagnosis or even the least likely. Of course more than one answer may be possible. So what you could try is working out an answer before looking at the possible solutions.'

Sarah then finds that she knows the answers to many of the questions. By understanding the format she can avoid the 'confuser' answer.

Sarah and the mentor work through 20 questions. The mentor gets quite a few wrong, which helps to make Sarah feel better. The mentor added, 'My last piece of advice is to go with your intuition or guess. If you change your answers you will get a lower mark.'

After practising these papers, Sarah feels much more confident and passes her next EMI online exam.

Coaching students helps them gain confidence in their exams. Discovering that consultants have gaps in their knowledge gives them insights into senior doctors' vulnerability and so is a valuable additional part of their professional development. Exam failure may be a symptom of more serious underlying problems. Just as a patient will present to a GP with a trivial physical problem such as a sore throat when there is a much bigger underlying psychological problem, so students will present with study problems masking other difficulties.

Case story Caroline

....

Caroline comes for help with her study technique as she has failed an online EMI exam. After doing a practice paper she said, 'I just feel so tired all the time.'

Her mentor asked, 'Tired?'

Caroline replied, 'Yes, I have so much on my plate just now. I am behind with my rent, I can't afford to eat properly and I am not sleeping.'

'Would you like to tell me a bit more?'

'I have split up with my boyfriend who was sharing the flat. It's in my name so I am responsible for the rent. I have tried getting a flatmate but no luck so far. I am so worried. My parents can't afford to help.'

'There are special emergency grants that the medical school can offer to give short-term help. If you like, I can speak to the administrator and you can email her for an appointment to meet. You will need to take your bank statements to her. She is really helpful and there are funds available to help in genuine cases of hardship.'

'That would be great. Thank you.'

'With regard to your accommodation problem, here is the telephone number of Moira, the student accommodation officer. Please give her a ring and let her know your situation. She may have the names of students looking to share a flat.'

'Thanks. I will do that. What a relief!'

'Please email me and let me know what happens. I am sure that once you are less worried, your studying will improve, but if you want a bit more coaching please get in touch.'

....

Any underlying cause for the student to be struggling may present with exam failure or studying problems, so the mentor needs to have a genuine curiosity to find out what is really troubling the student or doctor. This curiosity is accompanied by a genuine wish to help the mentee with his or her problem and to offer follow-up.

___ Coaching tips

Students often become anxious in clinical exams such as objective structured clinical exams (OSCEs) The following are some useful coaching tips for OSCEs.[5]

'Alison's Tips' when taking a history and sitting an OSCE

- Try to be as natural as possible.

- If stuck think 'Ideas, Concerns, Expectations'. Often these open questions allow the patient to give you more history.

- If stuck try to recap where you are so far aloud to the patient. He or she will correct you if wrong and summarising may lead the patient to give you further information.

- Think before you go into the exam station. What specific questions might you want to ask about the condition?

- When reading through the information sheet for the OSCE station, think about what information is being conveyed in this station. Does it seem to be about gathering information from a patient to make a diagnosis, explaining results or breaking bad news? What are the examiners after?

- Know before you go in what problem you want to focus on but still demonstrate active listening.

- Read the question.

- Use positive thinking.

- Concentrate on the patient; ignore the examiner as best possible.

- Speak to the simulated patient rather than to the examiner (unless otherwise directed).

- Always introduce yourself.

- Ask open rather than closed questions.

- Be aware of the time limit.

- If you need to make notes to remind you of the structure of the history you can do this, but taking notes as you go along will hinder your history taking.

- Once you have completed a station forget about it and focus on the next station.

___ Performance anxiety

Some individuals are prone to incapacitating anxiety in situations of public exposure and competitive scrutiny such as during exams.[6] This form of anxiety is allied to 'stage fright'. Of course some 'exam nerves' are normal; this section refers to disabling anxiety that prevents the student from performing to the best of his or her ability. Performance anxiety is characterised by a fear of failure and it can arouse a feeling of panic that results from an exaggerated adrenergic drive. This causes reduced concentration, memory blocks and a loss of steadiness in hands and voice. Students are more inclined to suffer such panic attacks when involved in more complex tasks, such as in OSCEs or ward simulation tests.

Predisposing factors to performance anxiety

Pessimistic talk before exams, predicting that questions will be unfair or that certain examiners are bound to fail them, can also put students at risk of disabling anxiety. Students with perfectionist personality traits are more prone to performance anxiety as they are less tolerant of making mistakes. In clinical exams and vivas some things are bound to go wrong and perfectionists find their performance suffers as they ruminate on their errors. Any situation that increases a perfectionist's sense of threat can precipitate performance anxiety. They might be apprehensive of failing to meet the examiners' expectations or overestimate the probability of failure. Being on one's own exacerbates performance anxiety as does a close proximity to the examiner. The student's perception of the examiner is also crucial; most examiners are not 'out to humiliate' students or to fail them.

Case story Esther

Esther is a final-year student who has never failed an exam but is very anxious about the ward simulation exercise. In this test she has to work as a Foundation Doctor in a simulated ward situation and is videoed. As she is doing the test she is being watched by two doctors on monitors who mark her performance. The test involves a handover from a registrar, interruptions to clerking a patient, prescribing, answering the telephone and dealing with a serious emergency – all occurring within 15 minutes. Esther has just learned she failed her first test and has a chance to repeat the test.

Esther says she is fine on the wards and enjoys doing shifts on the acute admissions unit in the hospital. She hates being filmed and is terrified she is going to make a mess of the test again.

The mentor sits down with Esther and they go through her video. They look at what went well and he also focuses on the moment when she became aware of the camera and 'froze'.

He asks if she can tell him a little more of why she hates being filmed. Esther says she has always been conscious of a birthmark on her face, which although very small is unsightly to her.

The mentor suggests that she try forgetting about the filming and just pretend she is on the acute admissions unit while taking the test. Esther also should brush up on her emergency drug prescribing. He also offers to make a note on her student file explaining her fear of the camera, in case the second test does not go well.

Esther is relieved and agrees to this plan, and passes her second ward simulation test.

Managing performance anxiety

The key to managing performance anxiety is to be prepared for the situation. Part of such preparation is for the student to accept that he or she will experience some anxiety and that this is necessary for an excellent performance. Preparation involves practice. It is surprising how many students will go to their finals viva without having had a practice viva and feedback from a mentor or tutor.

In the exam, students should be encouraged to try to forget about possible outcomes, focusing on the moment. They must be ready to carry out the tasks without evaluating themselves as they go along. For instance, in an OSCE, taking a history from the simulated patient involves thinking of the patient's problems rather than their own anxieties. In the unlikely event of an examiner asking an unfair question that embarrasses the student, he or she needs to pause and to reflect that no single examiner ever has the power to determine the result of an exam. It is much more important for students to admit they do not know the answer and to retain a calm demeanour and concentrate on the next question. Coming to the exam in the right state of mind means preparing oneself to feel physically fit by hydrating well, taking some exercise and using any relaxation techniques that have proven useful in the past. These might be visualisation, muscle relaxation exercises, breathing exercises or mindfulness mediation. A mentor might suggest some of the following tips for managing performance anxiety:

TIPS FOR MANAGING PERFORMANCE ANXIETY

- Focus on the moment.

- Forget the result.

- Do not judge your own performance.

- Do not guess the examiner's reaction.

- Do not aim for perfection.

- Self-acceptance rather than self-doubt.

- You will make mistakes, so stay focused.

- Eliminate images of negative possibilities.

- Hold performance in perspective.

___ Conclusion

Examiners want their students to pass exams but have a responsibility to ensure that high professional standards are maintained. It may help students to reflect that exams are not solely about their performance; they are also a measure of how well the institution has taught them. A mentor needs to keep in mind that students who come for help with exam anxiety may have other issues in their lives.

Key points

Exam anxiety is a common source of stress.

Mentors can help students by adopting a coaching role.

Students can be helped to overcome performance anxiety.

___ References

1 Robertson F, Donaldson C, Jarvis R, Jeffrey D. How can an academic mentor improve support of tomorrow's doctors? *Scottish Universities Medical Journal* 2013: **2(2)**: 28–38.

2 Royal College of Psychiatrists. *Mental Health of Students in Higher Education*. College Report CR166. London: RCP, 2011.

3 McManus I C, Richards P, Winder B C, Sproston KA. Clinical experience, performance in final examinations, and learning style in medical students: prospective study. *British Medical Journal* 1998; **316(7128)**: 345–50.

4 Fraser S W, Greenhalgh T. Coping with complexity: educating for capability. *British Medical Journal* 2001; **323(7316)**: 799–803.

5 Gillan A. Personal communication.

6 Wilson G D, Roland D. Performance anxiety. In: R Pamcutt, G McPherson (eds), *The Science and Psychology of Music Performance*. New York: Oxford University Press, 2002.

HEALTH PROBLEMS 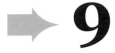 9

"Do you think you could do a locum at the Western?"
Prof. Marie Fallon

___ Introduction

The numbers and diversity of medical students have increased with the adoption of widening-access policies and a growing numbers of international students. Social changes such as higher rates of family breakdown and financial pressures affect the wellbeing of students. It is mental illness in students and doctors that is most often presented to mentors.

___ Mental health of students

Mental disorders exist on a spectrum of severity. At the severe end are illnesses such as schizophrenia, bipolar disorder, severe eating disorders, addictions and personality disorders. However, disorders at the less severe end of the spectrum, such as stress and anxiety, may still have an impact on the student's ability to complete coursework or pass exams. In recent years NHS mental health services have tended to concentrate on the needs of patients with more severe mental illness, bypassing those with less severe problems.[1]

The majority of students with mental disorders receive care from their GPs. Those with more severe psychiatric illness may be referred to specialist psychiatric services. Young adults between the ages of 18 and 25 are at high risk of developing serious mental illnesses such as schizophrenia and bipolar disorder.[1] In addition to primary care services, the university offers counselling services, but these need to be coordinated to provide effective care because students are forever on the move between home, university, main campus and outlying clinical attachments. In these situations, there is a risk that continuity of care breaks down and problems are missed.

Student counselling services are confidential and understand the connections between psychological and academic difficulties.[1] They do not diagnose or treat severe mental illness but are fully aware of when to refer to medical and psychiatric services.

Disability discrimination legislation, including the Special Educational Needs and Disability Act 2001, places a legal responsibility on universities for students with disabilities including those with severe or enduring mental illness.[1] The law stipulates that reasonable adjustments must be made to the study environment to compensate for disabilities and that there is a duty to promote equality of students and staff with disabilities. Any student with a diagnosed mental disorder may be eligible for Disabled Students' Allowance (DSA). This can help the student with the extra financial burdens of disability, including mental disorder and intellectual disabilities such as dyslexia.[1]

Some universities have mental health advisers who have qualifications in disciplines such as psychiatric nursing, occupational therapy, social work or psychology. They have the skills to assess how mental disorders in students may affect their learning.[1] They play a role in liaison between the university and NHS mental health services.

The commonest route into specialist NHS psychiatric care is by GP referral. Students should be encouraged to register with a local GP. However, because early intervention is advisable to prevent students dropping out, some universities have developed a 'fast track' service for acutely ill students.

Case story Monica

Monica, a fourth-year student, is referred to her mentor by a GP tutor as she had several days' absence and seems preoccupied and withdrawn. She has no previous mental health problems. The mentor sees her and asks Monica why she had been absent from the practice.

'I did not want to see patients', said Monica.

Silence.

Monica continues. 'You see, the voice inside tells me I am going to harm them. I keep hearing voices telling me to harm the patients. It's frightening.'

The mentor continues to listen and finds that Monica is feeling low and has paranoid delusions that her classmates want to poison her.

The mentor summarises. 'Monica, your GP tutor and I both want to help you. We realise that you are not well and need some help. You need to see your own GP today and have a break from your studies.'

'But I really want to be a doctor', replied Monica.

'Yes I know that and once you are well again you can get back to your course. Would you like me to speak to your GP and sort out an appointment for you?'

'OK, I know I am not right.'

The mentor speaks to Monica's GP who agrees that Monica needs urgent referral through the 'fast track'. An appointment is made for Monica with a consultant psychiatrist with an interest in student support for that afternoon. Monica is seen and diagnosed in the early stages of a paranoid psychotic episode and is admitted for assessment.

A major problem in helping students with mental illness is that NHS services are not usually adapted to the patterns of student life.[1] Students usually face lengthy waits for an appointment for clinical psychology or to see a psychiatrist. When the appointment arrives the student may be at home or in the middle of exams. In addition, treatment can be interrupted by vacation or attending blocks in hospitals distant from the main campus. In the case above the medical student's illness represented a threat not only to her safety but also to that of patients. The mentor's role is to ensure the student had rapid access to specialist services.

GPs are central in the management of mental disorders in students and usually liaise directly with counselling, mental health advisers or specialist psychiatric teams. Students may have difficulty in receiving continuity of care from a GP who knows them. When a student with a mental illness moves to a new location, details of his or her medication and medical history may not be transferred. There is, therefore, a need for closer collaboration between primary care and the universities; the requirement for confidentiality can complicate the transfer of information between them. Psychiatrists who are involved in the treatment of students may face a conflict of interest if there is concern that the student may pose a risk to patients. Any psychiatrist asked to assess the suitability of the student to continue with his or her studies should not also be responsible for treating the student.[1]

Students with mental health problems need enhanced academic and personal support because they are at a vulnerable transition between dependence and independence. Mentors and tutors should be able to recognise common mental disorders and those at risk of suicide. They should be aware too of the adverse effects of alcohol. Stigma surrounds mental illness, making it even harder for students and doctors to seek help.

In one study 29% of students described clinical levels of psychological distress; in 8% it was 'moderate to severe' or 'severe'.[2] In another study 9% of symptom-free students developed distress after two years at university, while 20% were troubled by anxiety.[3] Eating disorders are commoner in higher socioeconomic groups, with a peak onset in adolescence, making students particularly vulnerable. Students with autism spectrum disorders have difficulties with social interaction and coping with change; they may be at risk of depression, suicidal thoughts, anxiety and obsessive compulsive behaviours.[1]

___ Alcohol: the 'elephant in the room'

Many medical students drink alcohol to excess when free of constraints of life at home.[4] Although frank dependence is rare in young people, students are prone to harmful or hazardous drinking. In one university studied, only 11% of students did not drink alcohol. Of those who did 61% of men and 48% of women exceeded 'sensible limits' (21 units per week for men and 14 per week for women).[5] Hazardous drinking (>51 units per week for men, >36 units per week for women) was reported in 15% of those who drank alcohol and binge drinking occurred in 28%.[5] These high levels of alcohol abuse are of concern because they render a student vulnerable to ill health, academic underperformance and place them at risk of accidental harm and assault. There is also the significant risk that their alcohol consumption is the precursor of hazardous drinking with its risk of dependence in later life.[6] In another study 75% of medical students experienced alcohol-related 'provocation' during the previous year.[4] Commonly 'provocation' was coercion to drink an entire alcoholic beverage at once as part of a game. The provocation centred on three activities: peer–peer provocation during social activities, initiation rites and team-bonding activities.[4]

A mentor may need to explore the tension between the student's desire to 'fit in' with his or her peers, his or her attitudes to alcohol consumption and his or her developing identity as a doctor.[4] They need to be aware of signs of alcohol abuse and of local services to help students. The GP should be approached first by students with problem drinking. Students may also ask mentors for advice about coping with relatives who are abusing alcohol.

Universities should adopt a new approach to student induction and abandon the freshers' week binge.[1] Doctors have problems with excessive alcohol consumption and are three times more likely to die from cirrhosis than the general population. A large number of doctors brought before the General Medical Council (GMC) have problems with alcohol: 199 doctors out of 201 under supervision at the end of 2001 had problems with alcohol, drugs or mental illness.[4]

___ Drug misuse

At one university, cannabis was used by 22% of students once or twice, 23% more than once or twice and 17% of students were using it regularly. Three per cent of students were using ecstasy and/or amphetamines.[7]

___ Stress, compassion fatigue and burnout

Stress

Stress is a result of an imbalance between demands and coping resources.[8] Factors causing stress in doctors include: excessive workload, patients' suffering, medical errors, lack of support and poor leadership.[8] These factors can combine to create a sense of being overwhelmed. Poor coping strategies such as overworking or drinking heavily add to the problem. About 28% of doctors experience psychological distress compared with about 18% in the general working population.[9] Stress can lead to more serious consequences such as compassion fatigue and burnout as well as contributing to anxiety, depression and/or alcohol dependence.[8,10]

Case story **Juliet**

....

Juliet is a Foundation Doctor who is feeling low and finding it increasingly difficult to cope. One day she is sitting continuously answering her bleep, taking one phone call after another without having any time to carry out any of the requests or jobs. She feels she is a failure and leaves the ward in tears. She goes to her GP and tells her that she is not sleeping, worrying constantly about the work and has lost her appetite. She feels so bad letting her colleagues down. Her GP advises having some time off work and arranges for Juliet to see a counsellor.

PREVENTING STRESS

For students and doctors there are practical tips for preventing stress:

- find a mentor
- take exercise
- engage in reflection
- see family and friends
- manage your time
- use mindfulness meditation.

There are tips too for employers and educators:

STUDENTS

- encourage mentoring
- provide training in teamwork
- encourage students to ask for help.

DOCTORS

- have better supervision, induction and mentoring
- avoid sleep deprivation
- give time to reflect on challenging cases
- get informal support from family and friends.

Compassion fatigue

Compassion fatigue results from over-involvement in the doctor–patient relationship; it can be the result of caring for others in emotional distress without having appropriate support. Compassion fatigue may be similar to post-traumatic stress disorder (PTSD).[11] Compassion fatigue can lead to burnout. There are three main symptoms of compassion fatigue:[12]

1_ *Hyperarousal* – disturbed sleep, irritability, rage

2_ *Avoidance* – distancing from the patient; a desire to avoid thoughts and feelings associated with suffering

3_ *Re-experiencing* – intrusive thoughts or dreams and distress in response to reminders of clinical work.

Burnout

Burnout results from stresses in the workplace and results in poor patient care and medical errors.[12] Burnout can be caused by a sense of frustration, powerlessness and an inability to achieve work goals; it is particularly affected by the workplace culture. Excessive workload, lack of control, no rewards, no sense of community, and injustices can contribute to burnout.[12] A modern general practitioner only has limited time to do all the work he or she thinks should be achieved, but practice is messy and complex. Amery observes that, although we live in a relational, creative world, general practice is increasingly codified, stifling creativity with targets and tick-boxes, and with ever less room for GPs to express themselves. There is no time or space for a doctor to deal with the heavy emotional demands, to step back and to reflect on the work with a mentor.[13]

Case story Helen

Helen is a 35-year-old GP who is married and has three young children. For the past five years she has been a driving force in the practice, organising dispensing, arranging for students to be attached to the practice and attending local medical political meetings in the evenings. Her clinical interest is in palliative care and she works one session a week in the local children's hospice. She is respected and liked for her conscientiousness.

For the last six months her partners in the practice have become concerned by her behaviour. She is often late for surgeries and gives excuses for missing her evening meetings. She lost her temper with the practice pharmacist who had mislaid a repeat prescription. On two occasions she has asked the GP locum to cover her session at the children's hospice.

One morning Helen's husband rings the practice and says Helen has broken down in tears at home and says she cannot face coming into work any longer. He has requested Helen's own GP to come and see her at home.

Helen needed support earlier, but her GP partners were hesitant to ask her how she was coping; instead they denied there was a problem. Confronting colleagues about issues of performance is not easy. Instead she was allowed to become burnt out and had then to take a prolonged break from work.

Burnout is characterised by:

- emotional exhaustion
- depersonalisation (a feeling of detachment from the job)
- a sense of ineffectiveness.[14]

When emotionally exhausted the doctor makes efforts to cope by distancing him or herself from clinical work. Other signs of burnout include making negative comments about work, cynicism and avoiding the patient's suffering. Teams can also suffer burnout, which manifests as low morale, team conflicts, high job turnover and absenteeism.[14]

PREDISPOSING FACTORS

Highly motivated doctors with intense involvement in their work are at greatest risk of burnout.[12] Doubt, guilt and an exaggerated sense of responsibility drive these doctors to a destructive pattern of overwork. They neglect their family and outside interests to pursue their work goals. McManus *et al.* found that doctors with the greatest stress and emotional exhaustion had higher neuroticism scores and were more likely to prefer surface learning styles.[15] Lower conscientiousness also predicted greater stress, where the personality trait of agreeableness predicted a more supportive–receptive work environment. Their results suggest that a variety of approaches to work and the workplace climate result from differences in the doctors themselves as much as they do from differences in working conditions.[15] Engagement with one's job is the antithesis of burnout: it is characterised by involvement and efficacy in the workplace, a sense of competency and control in one's work.[12]

MEASURES THAT MAY PREVENT BURNOUT [12]

- Empathy and engagement.
- Mentoring and support.
- Narrative reflection.
- Sustainable workload.
- Control in the workplace.
- Rewards.
- Fairness at work.
- Mindfulness.
- Continuing education.

There is a misconception that being empathic with suffering patients must lead to emotional depletion. However, doctors who show true empathy are able to be highly attuned to the emotional distress of the patient. They try to see the world from the patient's perspective, yet at the same time retain their self-awareness and identity. Self-awareness permits the doctor to simultaneously attend to and monitor the needs of the patient, the work environment and his or her own subjective experience.[12] Paradoxically, when working with less self-awareness, the doctor is likely to lose perspective and experience more distress in his or her interactions with suffering patients. The doctor may mistakenly think empathy is a threat and so succumb to compassion fatigue or eventually burnout. Doctors with greater self-awareness suffer less as they will have a closer engagement, experiencing empathy as a mutually healing connection with their patients. Thus self-awareness can both enhance self-care and improve patient care. A doctor who adopts a self-awareness approach to self-care may remain emotionally available even in the most stressful clinical situations.[12] Two interesting approaches to enhancing self-awareness in students and doctors are mindfulness meditation and narrative reflection (Chapter 6).[12]

___ Mindfulness

Mindfulness is a heightened form of awareness of what is occurring in the present from moment to moment.[16] It involves becoming aware of our bodies and minds and our environment while remaining non-judgemental of what we observe. Mindfulness meditation helps with responding to life's challenges with a clear mind. This technique has been used in stress reduction clinics in the United States for both patients and doctors.[17]

___ Perfectionism

In some ways perfectionism is a form of self-harm and arrogance, as the individual cannot accept that he or she makes mistakes so sets him or herself up for failure. These students and doctors are under the delusion that they are able to achieve the unachievable. Perfectionism is neither skilful nor effective; although it is allied to conscientiousness, a positive personality trait for which medical students are selected, it can slip alarmingly into obsessive behaviour when the student is under stress.

___ Depression

Case story Adam

Adam is a fourth-year student who asks to see his mentor because he has missed a week of a clinical attachment in paediatrics. He tells the mentor that he is having great difficulty getting out of bed in the mornings. He just does not want to face the day. He wakes at 3 a.m. and lies in bed having morbid thoughts. He has never felt like this before and feels perplexed as to why this is happening to him.

His parents live 50 miles away and he only sees them every three months or so. He plays in the medical school football team but has lost interest in this activity.

The mentor listens to Adam's story and says, 'Correct me if I am wrong, but listening to you I get the impression you are feeling really depressed.'

Adam starts to weep silently.

The mentor said, 'It's OK to take your time. Have you felt so low that you are wondering whether it is worth going on?'

Adam nodded.

The mentor now has a clear picture that Adam needs to see his GP and that he can help by taking the pressure of work off his shoulders. 'Adam, the first priority is your health. You need to see your GP and have some help with your depression. You will need some time off but we can sort out how you will catch that up once you are feeling well again.'

The mentor sees Adam the following week and is disconcerted to find that he has not been to the see the GP. Adam explains that when he phoned at 9 a.m. he was told by the receptionist to try again the following morning as there were no appointments for the day. This has happened three days in succession. Adam then speaks to the triage nurse in the practice who tells him he should have been more assertive in the first place and insisted on speaking to the duty doctor. He would then have been seen straight away

The case story illustrates how difficult it can be for some patients to gain access to their GP. Many patients do not know how to navigate the complex appointment systems. As they do not want to be seen to bother the doctor they give up their efforts to make an appointment. The difficulty in making appointments with a GP is one of the many reasons why patients go to accident and emergency departments in hospital.

Adam was seen by his GP who arranged an urgent psychiatric assessment. He was advised by the psychiatrist to take some time off the course and to start a course of antidepressants.

Mentors do not have to make a diagnosis of clinical depression but they should be aware of the warning signs and refer the student or doctor to his or her GP if there is an indication that he or she may be depressed. If a student or colleague has experienced some of the following symptoms every day or nearly every day in the past four weeks it is time for a thorough assessment (based on the Patient Health Questionnaire-9 [PHQ-9]): [8,18]

- having little interest or pleasure in doing things

- feeling down, depressed or hopeless

- feeling tired or having little energy

- having trouble falling or staying asleep or sleeping too much

- having a poor appetite or overeating
- feeling bad about yourself
- having trouble concentrating
- moving or speaking slowly
- having thoughts that you would be better off dead or of hurting yourself.

If the mentor thinks the mentee is depressed, he or she should suggest an early assessment by the mentee's own GP. Commonly, students who develop depression will need a break from their studies and re-join their course the next year. If they have to leave the course temporarily, students should be reviewed regularly by their own GP or psychiatric services. They should also receive help and support in the period when they re-join the course. It is good for the tutor or mentor to maintain email contact while the student is away so that he or she does not feel isolated.

___ Suicide

The death of a young person by suicide is a tragedy. The annual suicide rate in England and Wales is 10/100,000 population and 17.3/100,000 in Scotland. The rates of student suicide mirror these rates. Between 1990 and 1999 there were 1482 student deaths from suicide in Great Britain.[19] Rates are highest in young males. Risk factors include social isolation, unemployment, depression, schizophrenia, drug and alcohol misuse, and a history of sexual abuse and self-harm.[19] Those responsible for providing support to students should ensure that they receive training in suicide risk assessment. This is a difficult area and students thought to be at risk should be referred for a thorough assessment, which should be carried out by counselling services, mental health services or in primary care. However, mentors and support tutors should be aware of the significance of depression and suicidal ideation, and feel confident about exploring these issues with students. Universities can provide more effective induction programmes and emphasise their wish for students to seek help if they are feeling depressed. Student counselling services, NHS mental health services, GPs and the university need to share their concerns, preferably with the student's consent. However, if there is a risk to life then they may disclose information in the student's best interests.

___ Eating disorders

Case story Rowena

Rowena is a second-year student with a history of self–harm. She has a regular appointment with a psychiatrist who monitors her bulimic eating disorder. Rowena lacks confidence, is perfectionistic and feels anxious. She is falling behind in her work and has failed two class assessments. She is referred by her psychiatrist to an eating disorder clinic but there is a three-month wait for treatment. Her psychiatrist advises a break from university to give the treatment the best chance by taking the pressure off Rowena. He says he will also arrange for her to have help from a clinical psychologist while she is at home.

She agrees to this plan but emails her mentor after three months saying she has heard nothing from the eating disorder clinic and has not had any follow-up from mental health services at her home. She is feeling low and her parents are worried about her lack of treatment. The mentor advises her to see her own GP and explain there has been a breakdown in communication. Her GP should contact her psychiatrist and arrange psychology support and find out what is happening to her eating disorder clinic booking. He asks Rowena to get back to him to let him know that arrangements have been made.

Problems in ensuring continuity of care are a recurrent theme in the care of students with mental health problems. The GP has a key role as a coordinator of care. Eating disorders are common and often undiagnosed in the student population.[20] Eisenberg *et al.* used a screening tool for eating disorders in a group of college students in the United States and found a prevalence of 13.5% in females and 3.6% in males. Of those identified by the screening with an eating disorder, less than 10% had been clinically diagnosed with an eating disorder. Twenty per cent of the students had received mental health treatment in the past year. An early diagnosis of eating disorders needs to be made as early treatment increases the chance of recovery. Students with eating disorders have higher risks of depression, anxiety, self-injury, substance misuse and suicidal ideation.[20] A large proportion of students with eating disorders are undiagnosed, being reluctant to seek help. A small but significant proportion of the students with eating disorders are male.

___ Other illness

This chapter has focused on mental health issues, which account for the great majority of health issues that students and doctors bring to a mentor. Medical students and doctors have a tendency to self-diagnose, self-medicate and present late after corridor consultations. Doctors are often reluctant to see their GP or take time off work. Students may be worried about confidentiality if they are being seen in local practices or in the teaching hospital. It may be helpful for students to consent to their clinical teachers being aware of a physical illness if it affects their attendance or studies.

___ Disability

A person has a disability when he or she has a physical or mental impairment that has a substantial and long-term adverse effect on that person's ability to carry out normal day-to-day activities.

The Disability Discrimination Act 1995 (DDA) required universities to make reasonable adjustments in the study environment to compensate students for their disabilities. They also have a positive duty to promote equality of students and staff with disabilities. It is unlawful for the university to discriminate against a person with a disability in terms of admission or by refusing to accept an application for admission.[1] Universities have Disabilities Services that are a source of information, help and support to disabled students. The mentor also has a role in improving the experience of students with disability, a role that is a shared responsibility of all staff, not just those with a remit for disability support.[1]

___ Conclusion

Mentors can play a central role in encouraging students or doctors with mental health problems to seek the appropriate professional help. They should be approachable and non-judgemental, giving plenty of time to assess the problem at the first meeting. This will build trust and let the mentee know that their problem is being taken seriously.

If the mental health problem is affecting the doctor's ability to practise then expert guidance must be sought on how to proceed. The medical defence organisations or the British Medical Association offer confidential, anonymous advice. The GMC may be contacted if patient safety is threatened.

The stigma of mental illness is still a major problem for doctors. The culture of invincibility in medicine is encouraged and vulnerability is denied. A culture shift is badly needed to acknowledge the emotional and psychological needs of students and doctors, and ensuring that every student and doctor has a mentor may be a good place to begin.[8]

Key points

There needs to be closer collaboration between universities and primary care with regard to mental health care of students.

Alcohol misuse is a major problem for many students and doctors.

Mentors could play a role in preventing stress and burnout.

____ References

1 Royal College of Psychiatrists. *Mental Health of Students in Higher Education*. College Report CR166. London: RCP, 2011.

2 Bewick B M, Gill J, Mulhern B, *et al*. Using electronic surveying to assess psychological distress within the UK university student population: a multi-site pilot investigation. *E-Journal of Applied Psychology* 2008; **4(2)**: 1–5.

3 Andrews B, Wilding J M. The relation of depression and anxiety to life-stress and achievement in students. *British Journal of Psychology* 2004; **95**: 509–21.

4 Black L F, Monrouxe L V. 'Being sick a lot, often on each other': students' alcohol-related provocation. *Medical Education* 2014; **48(3)**: 268–79.

5 Webb E, Ashton C H, Kelly P, Kamali F. Alcohol and drug use in UK university students. *Lancet* 1996; **348(9032)**: 922–5.

6 Moore R D, Mead L, Pearce T A. Youthful precursors of alcohol abuse in physicians. *American Journal of Medicine* 1990; **88(4)**: 332–6.

7 MacCall C, Callender J S, Irvine W, *et al*. Substance misuse, psychiatric disorder and parental relationships in patients attending a student health service. *International Journal of Psychiatry in Clinical Practice* 2001; **7(4)**: 137–43.

8 Iversen A, Rushforth B, Forrest K. How to handle stress and look after your health. *British Medical Journal* 2009; **338**: b1368.

9 Wall T D, Bolden R I, Borrill C S, *et al*. Minor psychiatric disorder in NHS trust staff: occupational and gender differences. *British Journal of Psychiatry* 1997; **171**: 519–23.

10 Hawkton K, Clements A, Sakarovitch C, *et al*. Suicide in doctors: a study of risk according to gender, seniority and specialty in medical practitioners in England and Wales 1979–1995. *Journal of Epidemiology and Community Health* 2001; **55(5)**: 296–300.

11 Figley C R (ed.). *Compassion Fatigue: coping with Secondary Traumatic Stress Disorder in those who treat the traumatized*. New York, NY: Brunner/Mazel, 1995.

12 Kearney M K, Weininger R B, Vachon M, *et al*. Self-care of physicians caring for patients at the end of life. *Journal of the American Medical Association* 2009; **301(11)**: 1155–64.

13 Amery J. *The Integrated Practitioner: surviving and thriving in health practice*. London: Radcliffe Publishing, 2014.

14 Maslach C. Job burnout: new directions in research and intervention. *Current Directions in Psychological Science* 2003; **12(5)**: 189–92.

15 McManus I C, Keeling A, Paice E. Stress, burnout and doctors' attitude to work are determined by personality and learning style: a twelve year longitudinal study of UK medical graduates. *BMC Medicine* 2004; **2**: 29.

16 Elliston P. Mindfulness in medicine and everyday life. *BMJ Career Focus* 2001; **323**: 2–3.

17 Kabat-Zinn J. *Full Catastrophe Living*. New York, NY: Delta, 1990.

18 Kroenke K, Spitzer R L, Williams J B. The PHQ-9:validity of a brief depression severity measure. *Journal of General Internal Medicine* 2001; **16(9)**: 606–13.

19 Universities U K. *Reducing the Risk of Student Suicide: issues and responses for higher education institutions*. London: Universities UK, 2002, www.healthyuniversities. ac.uk/uploads/files/uuk_scop_report__reducing_risk_of_student_suicide.pdf [accessed 25 June 2014].

20 Eisenberg D, Nickett E J, Roeder K, *et al*. Eating disorder symptoms among college students: prevalence, resistance, correlates and treatment-seeking. *Journal of American College Health* 2011; **59(8)**: 700–7.

PSYCHOSOCIAL ISSUES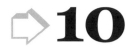

"Microbiology would be an interesting BSc. There is a doctor working on pyocines ... "

Prof. Gerry Collee, advising on a choice of research projects

___ Introduction

Students and doctors, like patients, bring problems that are influenced by their social and cultural setting. This chapter looks at the issues that may affect special groups of students and doctors: widening-access students, overseas students and doctors, graduate students and locum and out-of-hours GPs. The way in which bereavement can have an impact on the student's or doctor's work is explored. Financial and family problems that affect the student's or doctor's work will be explored. Finally, there is a note on social networking.

___ Widening-access students

Students from sectors of society that traditionally do not participate in higher education are admitted under widening-access policies. Universities have been encouraged to adopt inclusive strategies by financial incentives. While the widening participation has enriched medical schools by increasing diversity, these students often need support, particularly in areas of the 'hidden curriculum'. There is a clear link between lower socioeconomic status and dropping out.[1]

Case story **Stephen**

Stephen is a first-year student and part of a group of six widening-access medical students. He attends the group meeting each semester with their mentor. During these meetings the students set an agenda for topics they wish to cover. Each student gives a five minute presentation on the topic, and the rest of the group give feedback. Topics include the GMC's *Tomorrow's Doctors*, the hidden curriculum, failure and ethical dilemmas.[2]

Today's topic is failure. Each member of the group begins by describing a failure that he or she has experienced and the feelings it aroused in him or her. The mentor begins by picking out a rejection letter from the editor of a medical journal. The group discuss the feedback in the letter and comment on the positive and negative aspects. The lesson learned is that if you do not submit work it will not get published. The mentor comments on famous rejections such as Agatha Christie who had dozens of refusals of her first Poirot novel. From the discussion the students gain self-confidence and see that failures can have positive consequences, and that they are not reflections of their worth but an integral part of learning.

Group mentoring can be effective in covering issues that affect all members of the group.

A trusting environment is ensured by adhering to the ground rules (Chapter 2). The mentor explains that each member of the group can come to see him if there are individual problems he or she would like to raise. A group setting can be a good way of discussing the 'hidden curriculum', the process of becoming integrated into the medical community. Widening-access students, although academically bright, may not have the advantage of inside knowledge of the culture of medicine that students coming from medical families have grown up with.

Case story Stephen [continued]

After the meeting Stephen hangs behind and asks the mentor if he might have a private word.

He is concerned that one of his flatmates, a third-year dental student, is drinking heavily and encouraging the other members of the flat to go out every night to get drunk. The mentor asks Stephen if he knows the student well enough to suggest he gets some help from his GP or student counselling. Stephen is offered the telephone number for student counselling and told that his flatmate could just drop in to the counselling offices without making an appointment.

When a student comes to raise concerns about another student it is sometimes hard for a mentor to maintain confidentiality while still helping the troubled student. Mentoring and support are voluntary, and the student in difficulty has to take the first step and seek help.

___ Mentoring for overseas doctors [3,4]

International students come from a wide range of cultural, ethnic and religious backgrounds.[5] In considering their support the mentor needs to be aware of the additional challenges they face in adjusting to living and studying in the UK. They may be unable to afford regular visits home and may lack English language skills. They, and their families, have high expectations of academic success and may be under pressure because their parents are funding them.

Lingam and Gupta describe a mentoring scheme that aims to identify career goals, assess educational needs and develop an action plan.[3] The mentor helps doctors to achieve their professional goals by advising on cultural and communication issues, CVs and research. The mentor helps his or her mentee to understand the politics and organisation of UK medicine. He or she can advise on appropriate behaviour in different situations and offer time to debate values and ethical problems. With such support the mentee can enjoy the challenge of the changed environment and develop a flexible attitude to learning.

Case story Kim

Kim is a third-year medical student and comes from Hong Kong. She meets the mentor after failing an online exam. During the meeting to discuss her learning styles Kim reveals that she is doing medicine just to please her parents. 'As soon as I finish my degree I will look for a post in journalism as I really want to be a reporter.'

Her mentor asked her which parts of the course interested her. Kim said she enjoyed practical subjects such as surgery. The mentor listened and helped Kim to understand the strategy of answering online multiple-choice exams.

Two years later Kim returned asking for a practice finals viva. The mentor asked how she was getting on and Kim was full of enthusiasm for her Foundation Year posts. The mentor asked what had happened to enthuse her so much about medicine. 'I enjoyed seeing patients so much and particularly liked general practice. It is amazing that I ever considered giving up medicine. I now know it's what I really want to do.'

Kim and her mentor spent some time discussing the career path to general practice.

___ Graduate students

Graduate-entry students account for nearly 10% of the UK medical school intake. With more life experience they contribute to increasing diversity in medical students and doctors.[5] In a study of struggling graduate students, Garrud and Yates concluded that they faced much the same issues as undergraduate students, but the range of problems may differ in quality.[6] Graduate students often have issues of balancing their work with a family and they may have financial problems. In addition, they may not wish to join in the largely alcohol-based social activities of their younger colleagues, which may lead to isolation and loneliness. However, with their maturity they can be a strong source of support to the undergraduate students, sometimes acting in a peer mentoring role.

___ Bereavement

It is not uncommon for students to be bereaved during their medical course. The university should be informed in order that appropriate adjustments to the student's course can be made. The mentor, or anyone supporting students, needs to be aware of the types of grief reaction and to be sensitive to the effects of grieving on the student's performance on the course.

___ Grieving

Normal grieving is a form of suffering with physical, psychological and social components. Emotional distress may be episodic and can involve crying, rumination about the deceased and the whole spectrum of emotions from anger, guilt, fear, anxiety to despair.[7]

Case story **Sara**

Sara is a GP registrar who lives alone. She is called out of her surgery to see two police officers who inform her that her mother has been killed in a road accident. Her GP educational supervisor, Mary, sits with her and offers to take her home when she is able to recover herself. Mary asks who Sara would like her to contact and then contacts her sister who lives in a nearby town. Sara tells Mary that their father died when they were children. Mary advises Sara to let her GP know what has happened and suggests that she stay away from work for the next fortnight at least. She gives Sara her home telephone and mobile, and tells her not to hesitate to call her if she would like to talk. Mary emphasises that Sara need not think about work: 'This is a time when you need to be with your sister and close friends.'

Sara comes back to the practice two weeks later, saying that she would prefer to be at work. She talks to Mary and says she is sad, not sleeping and often feels frightened that something terrible will happen to her sister. Mary listens to her and reassures her that these feelings of despair and fear are a normal part of grieving. Sara tells Mary of her distress when as a 12-year-old child her father died of renal failure and she was not allowed to go to his funeral. Over the following months Sara sees Mary every four weeks and also talks to her sister and a close friend. She is now able to carry out her practice commitments and is seeking a part-time post as a GP in the same town.

Physical expressions of grief may include: numbness, restlessness, loss of appetite, sleeplessness, weight loss and fatigue. The bereaved student or doctor may withdraw socially, then 'search' for the dead person and may find reminders; they experience more pain and repeat the cycle by retreating again. This cycle of seeking and retreating is known as the loss-restoration model of grieving.[8]

Grieving is a normal reaction but the mentor needs to be aware of the possibility of abnormal grieving. Warning signs of abnormal grieving are characterised by intense separation distress and persistent protest against the death. The following symptoms should arouse suspicion of abnormal grieving if they are experienced daily and persist for at least six months: [9]

- non-acceptance of the death
- feeling life is meaningless
- lack of trust
- anger
- pessimism
- inability to carry out daily activities.

Bereaved students or doctors who are isolated and lack support are more at risk of abnormal grief reactions. Worden's practical Tasks of Mourning can give a helpful framework for mentors to understand grieving. Grieving is a dynamic process not a linear one so the bereaved person may fluctuate between the four 'tasks'.[10]

Tasks of mourning [10]

1_ Accept the reality of the loss.

2_ Work through the pain.

3_ Adjust to the environment in which the deceased person is missing.

4_ Emotionally integrate the deceased and start to move on.

___ Financial issues

Students often have financial problems that can impact on their academic progress. They are usually reluctant to discuss these but if assured of confidentiality they may disclose their worries to a mentor. Overseas students whose parents are funding their place at around £30,000 per year may feel a huge pressure to succeed in their studies.

Case story **Diana**

Diana is a third-year student who has been doing well in her course. She is referred by a clinical tutor as she says she is unable to take an intercalated degree in pharmacology because she is short of funds.

Chatting to her mentor she talks about her interest in pharmacology and is sad that she cannot pursue this at present. When the mentor explores this Diana says, 'Well I can't afford it. All students are short of cash.' The mentor listens and Diana breaks down. 'My parents have divorced and they can't help me any more. I am broke. I don't even know how I will pay for the medical course. I am so tired. I am working nights at the superstore stacking shelves.'

Her mentor advises her to go to Financial Services at the university who are helpful to students in genuine hardship. The medical school also has an emergency fund and there may be bursaries she could apply for that would help her in the long term. Diana looks hesitant and the mentor explains that these funds are not a charity but something to which she may be entitled. She has a good record and commitment to medicine so may stand a good chance of a bursary to enable her to complete her studies.

Diana decides not to pursue an intercalated degree at this stage but receives a bursary that enables her to complete her medical course and to give up her night work at the superstore.

Student mentors need contacts in the Medical School Office, Accommodation Services and the Student Finance Department so that he or she can refer students in difficulty. There is much greater chance of the student receiving help if there is a personal contact rather than an anonymous email to a department.

___ Family issues

Students are grown-ups and as such are entitled to complete confidentiality. Some parents find this difficult to appreciate and will phone or email a mentor with concerns about their son or daughter. The mentor must explain that they cannot discuss any student with their parents but they are prepared to listen to a concern. Family problems such as illness, separation, divorce, alcoholism, redundancy and bereavement can all impact on a student's performance.

Case story **Finlay**

Finlay is a fourth-year student who fails an OSCE for the first time. During feedback from his mentor, Finlay reveals that his father, who is terminally ill, is in a hospice 100 miles away and he is travelling home every weekend to see him. This has reduced his time for study and he finds it harder to concentrate on his work, but he has not told the medical school about this. The mentor asks what help Finlay needs.

Finlay says, 'It would be great to have a couple of weeks at home, Dad is dying and Mum needs the support.' With Finlay's consent the mentor speaks to the Teaching Dean who emails Finlay, expresses his concern and reassures him he can take four weeks away and still catch up with his course, but not to worry at present about his studies and be with his family.

When doctors listen to patients and take a history, the social context of the patient is understood to be important. Similarly, a mentor needs to appreciate a student's or doctor's family background if he or she is to gain a grasp of the problem. A struggling doctor or student, like a patient, rarely comes with a single issue; a mentor has to explore all the domains to gain understanding of the reasons for the difficulty. It is often only when issues are explored in depth with the mentee that the reasons for the poor performance become apparent.

___ Social networking

The majority of medical students and many young doctors use social networking sites such as Facebook. This has resulted in new ethical dilemmas in the tension between the personal and the professional.[11]

Case story Theo

Theo, a final-year student, comes to see his mentor for advice on his Foundation Year application. His mentor has been told in a conversation with another student about Theo's 'hilarious' Facebook page in which he has shared a holiday picture of himself standing on a table in a bar in Spain with a prawn up each nostril. The conversation comes around to social networking and the mentor tells Theo that some of his year found his Facebook page very funny. Theo is surprised. 'How did they get to see it? I thought the page was only open to my friends that I had accepted.'

Theo looked up his page with the mentor and found that he had not applied the correct privacy settings. He agreed that the picture did not present him as a reliable professional and realised that he should pay attention to conservative privacy settings and that in addition to his personal Facebook page he should have a professional page limited to contact details and interests.

Students have a right to privacy and protection from intrusion into their private lives, but social networking can create problems for them as professionals. There is a lack of awareness of the need for conservative privacy settings and the need for vigilance in monitoring their online presence.[11] When students make the transition to become doctors their new professional responsibilities may demand some modification in their online behaviour. Their online identity, particularly photographs, can have an impact on their professional relationships. Students and doctors must protect patient confidentiality. Doctors should never have a patient as an online friend. Students and doctors need to reflect on the risks and benefits of self-disclosure in social media.[12]

___ Conclusion

Social and cultural issues have an impact on most of the problems mentees come to discuss with their mentor. If problems are to be addressed effectively it is important to be familiar with the background of the student or doctor. It is sometimes surprising how much 'baggage' a mentee brings to his or her work. Often the role of the mentor in these situations is to be a listening ear, to give time and space to allow the doctor to express grief or other distress.

Key points

Widening-access and international students have increased diversity.

Grieving needs time and space.

Social networking can threaten professionalism.

Mentors need an effective network of contacts in generic support services.

____ **References**

1   Smith J, Naylor R. Determinants of degree performance in UK universities: a statistical analysis of the 1993 student cohort. *Oxford Bulletin of Economics and Statistics* 2001: **63(1)**; 29–60.

2   General Medical Council. *Tomorrow's Doctors*. London: GMC, 2009.

3   Lingam S, Gupta R. Mentoring for overseas doctors. *British Medical Journal* 1998; **317**: S2–7151.

4   Royal College of Psychiatrists. *Mental Health of Students in Higher Education*. College Report CR166. London: RCP, 2011.

5   Haldane T, Shehmar M, Macdougall C F, *et al*. Predicting success in graduate entry medical students undertaking graduate entry medical programs. *Medical Teacher* 2012; **34(8)**: 659–64.

6   Garrud P, Yates J. Profiling strugglers in a graduate-entry medicine course at Nottingham: a retrospective case study. *BMC Medical Education* 2012; **12**: 124.

7   Jeffrey E, Jeffrey D. *Enhancing Compassion in End-of Life Care Through Drama: the silent treatment*. London: Radcliffe Publishing, 2013.

8   Strobe M, Schut H. The dual process model of coping with bereavement: rationale and description. *Death Studies* 1999; **23(3)**: 197–224

9   Kissane D W, Zaider T. Bereavement. In: G Hanks, N Cherny, N Christakis, *et al*. (eds), *Oxford Textbook of Palliative Medicine* (fourth edn). Oxford: Oxford University Press, 2010, pp. 1483–501.

10 Worden W. *Grief Counselling and Grief Therapy: a handbook for the mental health practitioner*. New York, NY: Springer, 1982.

11 Lie D, Trial J, Schaff P, *et al*. 'Being the best we can be': medical students' reflection on physician responsibility in the social media era. *Academic Medicine* 2013; **88(2)**: 240–5.

12 Guseh J S II, Brendel R W, Brendel D H. Medical professionalism in the age of online social networking. *Journal of Medical Ethics* 2009; **35(9)**: 584–6.

WORKPLACE DIFFICULTIES 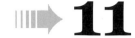 11

"Has there been a change in the patient's mood?"
Dr Huw Richards, psychiatry outpatient clinic

___ Introduction

Bullying and harassment arc among the biggest problems facing medical students and doctors in the workplace. This chapter also explores how a mentor might help an established GP with problems related to his or her workload and coping with the 'heartsink' patient. Teamwork is a part of modern medical care, but teams, like individuals, can suffer from burnout. The input of a facilitator can sometimes help doctors to improve their team-working skills.

___ Bullying and harassment

Bullying is persistent behaviour against an individual that is intimidating, degrading, offensive or malicious. It undermines the confidence and self-esteem of the recipient.[1] Harassment may be persistent or it may be an isolated incident. It is behaviour that might be related to a person's age, sex, race, disability, religion or sexuality. Harassment can take many forms: unwanted physical contact, inappropriate sexual advances, offensive emails or an invasion of privacy such as stalking.[2]

Bullying and harassment are widespread in the NHS and are the cause of 50% of stress-related workplace illness.[2] The reported prevalence of bullying in the workplace depends on how it is defined, but if a person feels bullied then bullying is taking place. Paice and Smith report a prevalence of 9.7% of trainees reporting bullying in the previous year.[1] Other reports give different figures: Frank *et al.* reports that 85% of medical students in the United States have been harassed or belittled during their training, with 13% describing severe incidents of bullying.[3] The General Medical Council's National Training Survey in 2013 reported that 13% of responding doctors in training reported being bullied during their training.[4] It seems that female doctors and those from ethnic minorities are most at risk. It is depressing that the figures are the same for those in 2013, showing that bullying is still a persistent problem despite NHS organisations professing a 'zero tolerance' to bullying.[4]

Not only does bullying have an impact on staff health and performance but it also jeopardises patient care; bullying is a patient safety issue.[1] If a mentor is told about bullying he or she must act to support the student or trainee. Challenging bullying in the NHS is often a traumatic experience for the victim and can also be stressful for those who support her.

Case story Fiona

Fiona is a Year Two specialist trainee doctor in a busy medical ward. Her consultant and educational supervisor persistently criticises her and makes sarcastic comments, usually on the ward round in front of the rest of the team. Fiona comes to see her mentor, saying that she is anxious, has lost confidence and feels low.

Her mentor Mairi asks Fiona what is wrong. Fiona says she has been to her GP because she has lost her appetite, feels lethargic and has palpitations on going to work in the ward. Her GP gave her mild antidepressants but Fiona has not taken them.

Mairi sits and listens. Fiona asked, 'Is our conversation confidential?'

Mairi reassures her and encourages her to share what is worrying her.

Fiona takes out an exercise book in which she has listed the dates and incidents where she feels she has been intimidated and humiliated on the ward by her consultant. 'I feel so low I just wonder whether it is worth going on. Yesterday I was having a three-month appraisal and he swore at me and said I was lazy and did not know enough. I burst into tears and he sneered at me, "You women just aren't tough enough for medicine".'

Mairi said, 'That sounds awful for you. Have you told anyone about this, Fiona?'

'I spoke to one of my friends who is a trainee in orthopaedics. She said everyone knows that this particular consultant is a bully and picks on females. Apparently it's not just me.'

Mairi asked, 'Has anyone made a complaint about his behaviour?'

'I gather not ... the trainees feel they will not be believed and that they will be labelled as troublemakers and not given a good reference.'

'Look Fiona, I can see from your notes that you have been persistently bullied. This is unacceptable. I know standing up to a bully is difficult but I can help you if you wish.'

Fiona said, 'What can I do?'

Mairi replied, 'Are you a member of the BMA?'

'Yes.'

'Well what I advise is that you speak to the local BMA adviser and to your deanery specialty adviser. It is Dr Shona Matheson and this is her phone number. I want you to get back to me once they have advised you and let me know.'

Three days later Fiona sees Mairi again.

Fiona said, 'The BMA adviser suggested I contact the hospital management and make a complaint. Shona said these cases were very difficult as it ends with my word against the consultant. She said it might be possible to get me transferred to another team. But I have done nothing wrong. I just don't understand why he picks on me.'

'I think when you contact the manager you should put your complaint in writing', replied Mairi. 'The hospital has a Dignity at Work policy that provides protection against bullying and harassment. They will then have to investigate this with a hearing, where you can choose to have someone with you.'

'Would you come with me, please?'

'Yes, but you might want more advice from the BMA. I am happy to read your letter to the hospital management. Please copy it to Shona at the deanery.'

'I will do it because I can't go on like this.'

Two weeks later Fiona says she has heard from the hospital management and the deanery and that they will put in place an investigation. She has to make a statement to her manager, who apologises that there is a huge backlog of complaints and that it will be two months before any hearing.

Mairi sees the manager and expresses her concerns that other trainees know that bullying is taking place but fear to do anything about it. The manager gets angry and warns Mairi that she should not be asking other trainees about this and that things might get very difficult for her. Mairi is taken aback by this intimidating reaction but gains some insight into the reasons why bullying largely goes unreported.

Two months later there is a hearing for Fiona who is accompanied by Mairi. At the end of the hearing the Medical Director tells Fiona she will be informed of their decision once they have interviewed the consultant.

Three weeks later the consultant goes on sick leave. Fiona receives a letter from the Medical Director informing her that her complaints have been upheld and apologises for the behaviour of the consultant, who is now on sick leave. He will be required to receive communication skills training on his return to the unit.

Fiona has a new educational supervisor and is much happier at work.

This story illustrates that it is not easy for students and trainees who are being bullied to seek support. The reasons for this are: [2]

- a belief that it will only make things worse
- a conviction that nothing will be done
- concerns about confidentiality
- fears of victimisation
- a fear of being labelled a troublemaker
- it will be seen as a failure.

Consultants who are stressed may take it out on junior colleagues; there may be a workplace macho culture where bullying is acceptable. If medical students experience bullying from negative role models there is a risk they will behave in that way when they become consultants. In the 'survival of the fittest' culture of certain parts of the NHS it is possible for bullying to go unreported. [2]

What needs to be done to stop bullying of students ___ and staff?

NHS employers need to have policies and procedures in place to deal effectively with cases of bullying and a determination to implement them. Managers and senior staff should ensure that staff can express concerns about bullying without fear of any reprisal and that victims of bullying receive support. Change is most likely to be effective at an organisational level; training should help staff to develop empathy for students and doctors in training. Senior staff who are humiliating juniors should be reprimanded and receive remedial training in communication skills. [5] The level of management support to employees is linked to levels of psychological distress and workplace bullying. Managers should take a stand against bullying and act as positive role models. [5] There needs to be an effective zero tolerance approach to bullying and harassment in the workplace. Consultants should receive 360° feedback from other members of the team; any suggestion of bullying should be dealt with by the trust medical director or relevant employer. Where there is a culture of bullying then training should be provided to foster proper professional working relationships and good teamwork.

Mentors and supervisors need to be alert to the possibility of bullying and ask students or doctors who seem unhappy, anxious or withdrawn whether they are being bullied. They should be ready to report doctors who teach by humiliation to the teaching dean in the university. In this way mentors can play their part in changing the current culture in the NHS, which tends to turn a blind eye to bullying.

___ Sharing the workload

Working in general practice has become more stressful; the specialty now faces a recruitment crisis. The rise in patient expectations and the increase in the size of group practices have increased the complexity of practice. Workloads have increased and many GPs do not feel that they have control of their work patterns. If a general practitioner feels that his or her workload is greater than that of colleagues he or she may become resentful and stressed.[6]

Case story Brian

Brian is a 45-year-old principal in an urban group practice of ten doctors. He has lost his enthusiasm for his work, finds practice meetings tedious and has become cynical about primary care. His desktop computer registers the years, months and days until his retirement. He comes to meet his mentor Peter who is a GP in another town. He tells Peter that he is fed up with primary care.

Peter asks him what has made him feel like this. Brian says, 'I am tired of having all the challenging patients, the ones with psychological problems, leading to longer consultations. Some of the partners finish their surgeries an hour before me, they leave for home on the dot at 6 p.m. and take their half-day at noon without fail. It is beginning to get me down.'

Peter asked, 'Down ... ?'

'Yes', replied Brian, 'I find I am not sleeping and having a whisky in the evenings. Pat and I don't go out much now. I am just too tired when I get home, I just want to eat and go to sleep.'

Peter went on. 'How long has this been going on?'

'I think things have got worse over the last three months.'

'How do you think you could address the workload issue?'

Brian replied, 'There are two other partners who feel fed up with the "fast consulters" who just get through the patient numbers and dash off home. I have chatted to them but they don't want to raise it in a practice meeting. They feel it might lead to divisions and make things worse.'

'Do you get on well with the other doctors in the practice?'

'Fine, on a day-to-day basis, but I really resent some of them because I am having to work harder seeing the stressful patients.'

Peter continued. 'Why not have a word about your concerns to your practice manager and ask whether she has any ideas for a fair allocation of work? Perhaps she might put working patterns down as an agenda item for your meeting. That way it could be discussed in a neutral way and not as a personal issue.'

Brian took up Peter's suggestion. When he had a coffee with Amy the practice manager he raised the issue of different working patterns. Amy said it would be a good idea. She had complaints from the receptionists that some of the partners who finished quickly were aggrieved that they had to deal with the extra patients, phone calls and prescription queries while the slower partners had a more leisurely surgery.

At the practice meeting it was apparent that all the partners had wanted to raise the issue but had felt the subject was taboo. They agreed that with all the part-time and assistant doctors they had lost the chance to really voice their feelings. Amy suggested having an afternoon meeting devoted to the issue and getting a facilitator to run the session. Everyone agreed this was a good plan.

A month later the doctors had the meeting on a training afternoon. They were able to share their feelings and decided that they needed to 'lighten up' and be a bit more flexible. They recognised that developing their trust in each other was the most important goal for the good of the practice. Amy said she would present workload statistics at future meetings just to show how hard they were all working. Brian felt much happier that the issue was in the open and that it would be regularly reviewed.

Brian's dilemma is a common problem, but one rarely voiced for general practitioners. A mentor needs to listen and resist the temptation to enter a therapeutic relationship, which would be entirely inappropriate. He might ask a few questions to screen for the presence of clinical depression but if he had a suspicion that the doctor was depressed he would need to recommend referral to his own GP or to occupational health (see Chapter 9). Amy's intuition that the general practitioners needed to get together out of work and debate the issue proved to be the breakthrough to solving this issue.

___ Difficult patient and difficult doctor

Every GP will be able to imagine a 'difficult' patient. A 'difficult' patient may have some of the following characteristics: demanding, non-compliant, have no medical diagnosis, alcoholic, morbidly obese or have predominantly psychosocial issues.[7] The 'difficult' patient can cause a GP intense frustration, stress and even moral distress. Pressures of time and an increasing workload for GPs are only going to exacerbate the problem of interactions with these patients. In the past the focus of research has been on the 'difficult' patient sometimes described as a 'heartsink' patient.[8] However, recent work has looked at the doctor's part in the interaction; for instance in one study the greatest predictor of 'difficult patient' consultations was not the patient but the doctor.[9] Doctors with poorer psychosocial skills averaged 28% difficult consultations whereas their colleagues who were more comfortable with dealing with psychosocial issues only reported 8% of consultations as 'difficult'. In another study the following common themes were identified among doctors reporting high levels of frustration: working more than 55 hours per week, depression and anxiety, larger number of patients with psychosocial problems or substance misuse.[10] What is clear from the research is that, as with the patient, the doctor brings his or her psychological and emotional baggage to the consultation.

Case story Tony, a GP

Tony groaned as he looked at the schedule for his Monday morning surgery. Mrs Boswell was coming in to see him again. He had seen her twice last week and almost every week or two for the past six months.

Mrs Boswell is a 32-year-old single mother of two children aged six and four years. She is morbidly obese. She complains of shooting pains in the left side of her abdomen and passing lots of wind. She has been referred to a gastroenterologist, surgeon and gynaecologist over the past six months and investigated fully. No diagnosis has been reached. She has had medication for irritable bowel, depression and had a variety of analgesics. None of these interventions has had the least effect on her symptoms and she continues to come to the surgery to see her GP.

Tony can feel a sense of frustration and anger building up as she tells him what a terrible weekend she has had with her pain. In desperation he suggests referring her to the chronic pain service to see if they can help. There is a four-month wait to get an appointment.

In the meantime Tony prescribes another analgesic and feels a failure as he ushers Mrs Boswell out of the consulting room.

Doctors do not like feeling frustrated and helpless. A mentor can help a GP with these problems simply by giving time and space to reflect on the case and to discuss options for coping with the problem.

—— How can a mentor help?

Listen to the story

The mentor can begin by asking if there are any cases that are causing the GP any difficulties. The GP can then describe the case and be encouraged to express his or her emotions and feelings. When the discussion is focused on a clinical situation the GP may reveal more about how he or she feels than if asked directly about his or her worries.

Positive feedback

The mentor can acknowledge how well the GP has done to persevere with the difficult problem despite the frustrations.

Reframing

The mentor can help the GP to see the problem in a different way. Rather than focusing on the *patient* as difficult, the mentor can describe the *clinical situation* as difficult. For instance, 'How can one approach the problem of chronic undiagnosed pain?'

Curiosity

The mentor can encourage the GP to regain a clinical curiosity about the patient. What are the patient's Ideas, Concerns and Expectations about his or her illness?

Goals of the consultation

The goals are centred on the individual patient. What is best for this patient? How does the patient feel any suggested intervention fits in with his or her goals?

Learning

The mentor can encourage further learning about conditions such as borderline personality disorder, alcoholism, obesity and management of chronic pain.

Support

There is an opportunity to support the doctor, listen to his or her concerns, acknowledge how difficult this is for the doctor and offer time in future to discuss these issues.

Set realistic goals

Agree some goals that are realistic which might help the doctor to cope better with these difficult patients, perhaps using the framework above.

Case story **Mrs Boswell**

Tony agreed that when Mrs Boswell returned he would begin the consultation by exploring her Ideas, Concerns and Expectations of treatment. He would also ask her how she was coping on her own and how her children were getting on. After summarising the problems he would try to involve Mrs Boswell in setting some treatment goals together, which would fit better with her expectations. After chatting to his mentor Tony also could appreciate that he found dealing with psychological problems most challenging. He was grateful for the feedback and was looking forward to seeing how these ideas might help Mrs Boswell.

The intervention of a third party, in this case a mentor, gives an opportunity to take a fresh look at these situations. GPs are under great pressure at present with an escalating workload and with targets to achieve. Support from a mentor would allow GPs to express their frustration and concerns, and receive positive feedback about their good work.

___ Conclusions

The examples discussed show that a mentor can play a helpful role in different ways. In challenging bullying a mentor acts as the young doctor's advocate. When helping an experienced colleague vent frustration about his or her partners the mentor adopts a listening role. It is helpful if a mentor has experienced these problems him or herself as this makes it easier to empathise with the distressed doctor. Finally, a mentor can act as a clinical colleague in debating the management of a difficult patient. In the course of these discussions the doctor being supported gains trust in the mentor. Consequently the doctor then feels safe to disclose some of his or her feelings and vulnerabilities. It is at this point where mentors can make their most helpful contribution to supporting a colleague. The alternative unsatisfactory outcome is to see a doctor's performance deteriorate whilst his colleagues do nothing. Mentoring as an accepted part of professional practice for all doctors would prevent this sad outcome.

Key points

Bullying should not be tolerated.

Problems between partners can cause a great deal of stress.

Clinical discussions can be a useful forum for exploring the doctor's real concerns.

Mentoring could help GPs before their performance resulted in complaints.

____ References

1   Paice E, Smith D. Bullying of trainees is a patient safety issue. *The Clinical Teacher* 2009; **6(1)**: 13–17.

2   Mistry M, Latoo J. Bullying: a growing workplace menace. *British Journal of Medical Practitioners* 2009; **2(1)**: 23–6.

3   Frank E, Carrera JS, Stratton T, *et al.* Experiences of belittlement and harassment and their correlates among medical students in the United States: longitudinal survey. *British Medical Journal* 2006; **333(7570)**: 682.

4   General Medical Council. *National Training Survey 2013: undermining.* London: GMC, 2013, www.gmc-uk.org/NTS_2013_autumn_report_undermining.pdf_54275779.pdf [accessed 25 June 2014].

5   Illing J C, Carter M, Thompson N J, *et al. Evidence Synthesis on the Occurrence, Causes, Consequences, Prevention and Management of Bullying and Harassing Behaviours to Inform Decision Making in the NHS.* London: HMSO, 2013, http://dro.dur.ac.uk/10533/1/10533.pdf?DDD45+DDC42+clfc44   [accessed 25 June 2014].

6   Branson R, Armstrong D. General practitioners' perceptions of sharing workload in group practices: qualitative study. *British Medical Journal* 2004; **329(7462)**: 381.

7   Abbot J. Difficult patients, difficult doctors: can consultants interrupt the 'blame game'? *American Journal of Bioethics* 2012; **12(5)**: 18–20.

8   O'Dowd T C. Five years of heartsink patients in general practice. *British Medical Journal* 1988; **297(6647)**: 528–30.

9   Jackson J L, Kroenke K. Difficult patient encounters in the ambulatory clinic: clinical predictors and outcomes. *Archives of Internal Medicine* 1999; **159(10)**: 1069–75.

10   Krebs E E, Garrett J M, Konrad T R. The difficult doctor? Characteristics of physicians who report frustration with patients: an analysis of survey data. *BMC Health Services Research* 2006; **6**: 128–36.

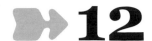

CHALLENGES

"You have to stop."

Dr Jim Moore, general practitioner

___ Introduction

Most of the book has described the virtues and benefits of mentoring for students, trainee doctors and general practitioners. However, mentoring, based on a close relationship, may become dysfunctional. This chapter examines what has been described as 'The Dark Side of Mentoring'.[1] Mentoring is usually a gentle, supportive process but sometimes the mentor has to act swiftly. This chapter covers some situations where a rapid response is required.

Problems can arise in any professional relationship, whether it is a doctor–patient relationship or a mentor–mentee relationship. Barriers to mentoring concern timing, logistics and 'personal chemistry'.[2] Problems can arise because the relationship is a strong emotional one and boundaries may be broken. There may also be personality clashes, cultural and gender issues, over-involvement or broken confidentiality. The mentor may have conflicting roles of manager or assessor or be constrained by workload from providing time for the mentee. Mentoring should not be involved with assessment or remediation, and should be voluntary.

Case story Anita

Anita, a Foundation Year 2 doctor has an educational supervisor and mentor, Prof. Green. Anita has a longstanding eating disorder and is prone to bouts of bulimia when under stress. She has found it difficult to cope with the workload on the medical unit and has begun to self-harm. She is unwilling to discuss this with her mentor because he is so busy and she is worried that he will not give her a good reference. Prof. Green mentors four young doctors and meets them in a group twice a year just to 'check that there are no problems'. Unsurprisingly perhaps, few problems are raised in the group, discussion being limited to tips around career progression.

___ Unsuccessful mentor–mentee relationships

Anita's story reflects several pitfalls of mentoring. The matching of mentor and mentee is critical. A mismatch may be due to personality clashes and/or gender issues. The young female doctor finds it impossible to discuss her self-harming with a confident male professor. He is only comfortable with a limited mentoring role and is not prepared to engage with emotional issues. In Anita's story there is a mismatch between the expectations of the two members in the relationship. Anita expects a mentor who will provide psychological support and Prof. Green sees his role as providing career advice. There is a lack of understanding on his part of the process of mentoring. Mentoring relies on a close, individual relationship and cannot be conducted satisfactorily by a brief twice-yearly group meeting to discuss career plans.

Mentors and managers may fail to understand the level of commitment involved in mentoring, which is a developing relationship requiring time. The process involves both mentor and mentee reflecting on the mentee's concerns and in this process the mentor helps the mentee to grow through self-discovery. Many senior clinicians who would like to be mentors lack the time to devote to this activity because meetings with the mentee clash with work commitments. This is an issue that affects the organisation, which should place a value on mentoring and devote the time and resources required so that it can be conducted effectively.

Recruitment of suitable mentors and providing them with training and support presents another challenge. There is a shortage of female mentors that puts pressure on the mentors in post, who may take on too many mentees in an effort to plug the gaps. Female members of minority ethnic groups who lack the choice of a female mentor may be reluctant to access a male mentor. Mentees who do not have a good relationship with a mentor may be jealous of colleagues who are in a successful mentoring partnership. If there is a personality clash it is much better for the mentee to choose another mentor because a relationship of mutual trust and respect is essential for mentoring to succeed.

Case story Megan

Megan is a 35-year-old general practitioner who was assigned a mentor after concerns were raised during her annual appraisal. The concerns related to the 360° feedback from practice staff who commented on her rather abrupt and dismissive manner. Megan did not find it easy to talk to her mentor, a 55-year-old male GP in another town. After two meetings Megan asked if it would be possible to have a female GP mentor and this was arranged for her.

Megan met her new mentor, a 40-year-old female GP, and was relieved to be able to discuss her difficulties, which related to her abusive husband.

Optimally mentees should always have a choice of mentor. Unfortunately this is not often practical and most mentor–mentee relationships work out well. However, if there is a real difficulty, such as in the case above, then the mentee should be allowed to opt out of the relationship.

___ Boundaries

If there is a lack of clarity of professional boundaries there is a risk that mentoring changes to become personal therapy. The mentor must remember that he or she is not the mentee's doctor and should not take on a therapeutic role. This can be difficult when listening to a bereaved student or to someone who is depressed if the mentor is clinically skilled in dealing with these issues. The mentor's role is to be aware of these possibilities and to refer the mentee to the proper agency. If there are no clear boundaries the mentor can become over-involved, taking on all the mentee's problems and trying to solve them alone.

Case story Alex

Alex is a clinical tutor in the university department of general practice. He has taken on a mentoring role for overseas students. Pankaj is a fourth-year student whose parents live in Chennai. Pankaj comes to see Alex for help with his study skills and in writing his portfolio. In the course of their second meeting Pankaj says that he has been falling behind in his studies and has been missing lectures. Alex comments, 'I can see from your student file at least you have been attending the clinical skills tutorials.'

Pankaj looks abashed. 'I have missed quite a few but my girlfriend Rita who is in my group has signed my name on the attendance sheet.'

Alex looks alarmed. 'But that is most unprofessional, I will have to raise this with the Dean.'

Pankaj replied, 'But you promised our conversations would be confidential. Please don't do anything to get Rita into trouble.'

'Look Pankaj, I need to think about this. Please come with Rita and see me tomorrow afternoon. I will not do anything in the meantime.'

Next day Rita and Pankaj come together to meet Alex.

Alex begins. 'Rita, Pankaj has told me that you have filled in his name on three attendance forms when he was in fact absent. Is this true?'

Rita bursts into floods of tears. 'We are in so much trouble, my parents are very poor and have been threatened by debt collectors. They live in London. Pankaj has taken time out to go and support them and to help them see a bank manager and someone from Citizens Advice. He was so worried that if he did not attend the tutorials he would not be allowed to sit the end of year exams.'

Alex felt so sorry for Rita and agreed to keep the matter confidential provided that it did not happen again. He missed an opportunity to point out that Rita was involved in fraud and this was a serious lapse of professionalism. He made no record of the conversation and did not take it further.

Three months later a tutor noticed that the attendance sheet did not match the attendees in a problem-based learning group. It was Pankaj who was absent and Rita who covered up for him again. When challenged Pankaj said he had told his mentor Alex in the past and nothing was done so he assumed it was permissible if he had good reasons.

Alex was asked to meet the teaching Dean and explain his actions. He reflected that he had become over-involved in Rita's and Pankaj's family problems, felt sorry for them and had tried to help by having an 'ostrich response', i.e. burying his head in the sand, and hoping things would settle. He realised this was a serious misjudgement and apologised for not taking proper action. The Dean saw Rita and Pankaj and gave them both a written warning, saying if there were any further serious lapses in their professionalism they would be referred to the student Fitness to Practise Committee. Pankaj was assigned a different mentor. The Dean suggested that Alex take a break from mentoring for a year.

This case illustrates the dangers of becoming over-involved in the mentee's problems and so losing perspective. The mentor had good intentions but was unwittingly drawn into a collusion with the student.

When working in a close relationship with students and doctors in training who are distressed, the mentor must be on his or her guard against unprofessional emotional attachment to the mentee. If at any time the mentor feels vulnerable to this they should either have another tutor with him or her in the meeting or assign the mentee to another mentor. For these reasons, although the room for the meeting is chosen to provide privacy, it should be readily accessible to other staff.

Poor mentoring relationships can result in the mentee being over-protected, creating an unhealthy dependency. In any close relationship there is a risk of sexual attraction and sexual overtones to the mentor meetings. This is unacceptable and represents serious professional misconduct on the mentor's part.

The mentor may be a poor teacher and role model, and it may not be helpful for the mentee to misguidedly copy the mentor's work style. Role modelling is effective in promoting professionalism only if the mentor is demonstrating good practice.

___ The challenging doctor

The student or trainee who lacks insight presents a particular challenge to mentoring. Insight is related to the motivation to engage in reflection but an individual will not necessarily gain insight merely by self-reflection. By using strategies such as role modelling and small-group work it is possible to move slowly towards a new stage. Here, the student or doctor who lacks insight can set aside blame and begin to take responsibility for his or her professional development.

Tips for mentoring the challenging doctor

Faced with a challenging trainee who lacks insight into his or her problems and relates poorly to colleagues and patients, the mentor should try to:

- listen
- seek evidence of insight, asking about the trainee's expectations, effect on patients and colleagues, and the reasons for his or her difficult behaviour
- remain supportive
- focus on the positive
- be non-judgemental
- encourage change and look for evidence of change in behaviour or mood
- identify common themes in the story, looking for the underlying problem and any extenuating circumstances
- encourage reflection by sharing stories (see Chapter 6)
- act as a role model
- give skilled, honest feedback as soon as possible after the event
- maintain confidentiality
- keep records.

In situations where patient safety is at risk, or where the doctor is a danger to him or herself, then referral to either the university or General Medical Council (GMC) becomes necessary. If there are mental health issues then Occupational Health or the mentee's GP will need to be informed.[3]

___ Unrealistic expectations and overload of mentees

An effective mentor may be instrumental in radically improving the lot of a struggling student or doctor. However, this success can generate further problems. The trainee or student may become over-dependent on the mentor and demand too much of their time. In such a situation another mentor might be better taking over the mentee, or the mentor should talk to a colleague about the way in which he or she is handling the mentee's problem. Another problem for successful mentors is that they get overwhelmed by mentees who choose to see them. This is an issue for the organisation to ensure an equitable allocation of mentees to each mentor.

___ Mentoring not valued by organisation

There are many strands to supporting students and doctors so it is often difficult to define the contribution of a mentor in a mentee's learning and professional development. Mentoring takes time and there is a cost to the organisation. However, if one looks at the cost of a failed medical student or a doctor who drops out of medicine then mentoring represents a good investment, not just financially but also in alleviating personal and psychological distress.

___ Conflict with colleagues

Acting as an advocate for a student can involve the mentor in challenging assessments of students or behaviour of colleagues.

Case story Patrick

Patrick, a fourth-year medical student, came to see his mentor. He had been asked to repeat a case assignment because the original was handed in two days late. He explained to the consultant marking the assignment that his grandfather had died in the week before the deadline for handing in the work. The consultant had appeared cynical and said, 'It's amazing how many grandparents die during the final two years of medical studies.'

The mentor listened and Patrick explained that his own father had died when he was seven and he had been brought up by his mother and her parents. He had been devastated by his grandfather's death. Patrick consented to the mentor speaking to the consultant.

The mentor saw the consultant and as soon as he understood the situation the consultant apologised to Patrick and agreed to mark the original work.

The mentor needs to have good working relationships with his or her colleagues and to have credibility and their trust. Listening to students and doctors in training, the mentor may hear stories of their colleagues behaving badly. The mentor should not just accept these at face value but continue to listen without ever making any derogatory comments about colleagues.

However, if a colleague is being unfair to a student then the mentor has a role in standing up for the mentee.

___ Workload

The mentor usually has a full clinical workload so allowing time for seeing students or doctors may be difficult. Mentoring requires continuity and an easy access for mentees. The methods of contact should be arranged on the first meeting and ground rules set for meeting frequency and length. It is dispiriting for students if they cannot arrange to see their mentor of if he or she does not respond to their emails.

___ Cultural and gender issues

It may be that certain cultural or gender issues would make it difficult or embarrassing for a student to discuss an issue with a mentor of the opposite gender. Female Muslim students might for example be reluctant to discuss relationship difficulties or self-harming with a male mentor.

Mentors should be sensitive to these possibilities and offer alternative support for the student or trainee.

___ Broken confidentiality

Confidentiality is the cornerstone of the trusting relationship and should not be broken unless there is a threat to the safety of patients, the mentee or others. It is important that the mentee sees and approves any written record made about him or her. Mentors should extend the same standards of confidentiality to colleagues that they are mentoring as they would to patients. If the mentor is keeping unofficial '*aide mémoires*', these should be anonymised, kept securely and destroyed once they are no longer needed. In 'off the record' conversations it is probably safest not to keep any record. Although confidentiality is key to the trust a mentee places in the mentor, it can place the mentor in a difficult situation. He or she has to explain at the outset that behaviour which threatens the safety of patients or of the mentee cannot be kept confidential. Criminal acts, drug and alcohol misuse, fraud and serious professional misconduct by the mentee have to be reported to the appropriate authority: police, university, employer or the GMC. Sometimes students and doctors are struggling with issues that, although not affecting patient safety, are affecting their performance, but are unwilling for the mentor to disclose the information. In these difficult situations, allowing a little time to pass may give the mentee space to develop trust in the mentor's judgement. For example, where there has been a family bereavement, the mentor can offer to speak to tutors or educational supervisors. It is also important that students and trainees are aware that counselling services provided by Occupational Health, the university or the deanery are confidential.

Problems can occur when mentors or tutors take on a therapeutic or a clinical assessment role. Crossing boundaries creates a conflict in roles. For example, if a psychiatrist is involved as a mentor or tutor for a student it is not appropriate that he or she should have an assessment or clinical role for that student.

The mentor's records may create confidentiality problems. It has been emphasised that documentation is important but a secure method is needed to store records of 'off the record' conversations. The mentor needs to have a secure form of *aide mémoire* of these 'off the record' conversations, often around highly sensitive issues.

Case study Belinda

Belinda is a specialist trainee in general practice and Fred is her educational supervisor and her mentor. He has heard from one of the partners in the practice that Belinda seems withdrawn and is sometimes short tempered. Fred decides to meet Belinda to review her GP attachment after three months. In the course of discussion on her progress she becomes tearful and asks if she can reveal something that she does not wish to go on her trainee record. Fred explains that as long as she has not done something criminal or it is not going to affect the safety of others her information can be kept completely confidential.

Belinda then breaks down and says that about six months ago a man tried to rape her. She has been to her own general practitioner who referred her to the hospital sexual health clinic and gave her the number of the local rape support service. Belinda was adamant she did not want the police involved. She had not been able to talk about the traumatic episode to anyone and she had not contacted the counselling service.

Fred asked about Belinda's relationship with her family. She asserts that she had always been close to both parents and to her younger sister, and she has a supportive boyfriend, whom she had known for three months, but did not feel she could talk to them. Belinda had not found the contact with the hospital clinic helpful; they just confirmed that she had not acquired a sexually transmitted disease and that she was not pregnant.

Fred expressed his sadness at hearing of this incident and reassured Belinda that he would not make any formal record of their conversation. He praised Belinda for her courage in raising the issue. It was clear that she needed someone to talk to about her traumatic experience. Indeed, Belinda said she would like to be able to talk to her mother but was worried about upsetting her. Fred asked when Belinda was next going to see her mother and suggested she should find a good moment when she could have a quiet, private discussion. Fred asked Belinda to reflect on a situation if the roles were reversed and it was her daughter who had been raped. Belinda said 'Of course I would want to help', and agreed she would speak to her mother at the weekend.

The supervisor advised contacting the police but Belinda was adamant that she wanted to put the incident behind her. He suggested that Belinda might also like to talk to a particular female counsellor in the deanery with expertise in this area. Anything she discussed would remain confidential. Belinda was keen to pursue this and Fred helped Belinda to arrange an appointment with the counsellor. The supervisor asked Belinda to keep in touch by email and they agreed to meet in a month for a review.

A tension can arise between maintaining confidentiality and accessing appropriate support for the mentee. If the mentee feels that information is to be shared he or she will be less likely to access support. In Belinda's case the supervisor felt that Belinda should talk to her mother and to the police, but she did not want to make a formal complaint to the police.

___ Advocacy

A mentor may need to act to support and advise a student, and help to present his or her case in the best possible light in situations of formal review such as Fitness to Practise hearings or when termination of the student's studies is possible. Acting as an advocate for a student requires diplomacy and negotiation with colleagues who may not be aware of all the issues behind a student's poor performance.

Case study Caroline

Caroline had narrowly failed her first-year exams and her resits. She came to the mentor, who asked about her study techniques. Caroline spent long hours copying out her lecture notes and trying to memorise them. She had never failed any exams at school and had achieved the highest grades in her A levels. She was highly conscientious and took great pains to check her work. Her family were supportive and she had made good friends at the university and her interests included drama and netball. She had wanted to be a doctor 'for as long as I can remember'. She asked the mentor to help her in her appeal to the university Academic Review Committee, who were meeting to decide whether to terminate her studies.

The mentor referred her to the Academic Study Skills department; here Caroline was helped to recognise that her perfectionistic personality was hampering her studying and shown more effective study techniques. The mentor wrote a letter supporting her application to repeat her first year of study. It explained to the committee the steps that Caroline was taking to make sure that she would pass if she was given another chance. Caroline and the mentor agreed a plan of regular review of her progress in the event of her appeal being successful.

Caroline was allowed to repeat the year as she only failed by the narrowest margin.

Mentors need to have credibility to ensure that their advice on behalf of students is considered by the faculty of medical school. Mentors can be involved in bringing about change not only in individuals but also in institutional systems of support.

___ Rapid responses

On rare occasions situations arise that demand a rapid response. Some of these situations have been covered in the preceding chapters. Examples of such mentoring 'emergencies' include:

Risk of suicide

The mentor should be aware of the factors that increase the risk of suicide: depression, other mental illness, negative life events, previous history of self-harm, alcohol or drug misuse, family history of suicide and access to methods of self-harm.[4] The main goal with a student or doctor who may be suicidal is to prevent suicide rather than achieve an accurate prediction. It is far better to be cautious and refer, and quite safe to ask about suicidal ideas. Other questions that should be raised include:[4]

- Are they feeling hopeless, or that life is not worth living?
- Have they made plans to end their life?
- Have they told anyone about it?
- Have they carried out any acts in anticipation of death (e.g. putting their affairs in order)?
- Do they have the means for a suicidal act?
- What support is available for them?

If the mentor feels there is a risk of suicide, the student or doctor should be referred urgently to his or her GP. The student or doctor will need to be informed in a supportive manner that he or she is a risk to him or herself, and so confidentiality of the relationship may be broken to act in the mentee's best interests.

Acute psychotic illness

The case of a student with an acute psychotic breakdown is described in Chapter 9. There may be a risk not only to the student or doctor but also to patient safety. Again, urgent referral to the GP is required and rapid psychiatric assessment will need to be arranged.

Rape

If the student or doctor alleges that there has been inappropriate sexual advances or rape then the mentor should ensure the individual records in writing the events that took place. The student should be advised to see a GP, attend a hospital sexual health clinic, inform the police and receive counselling from local rape counselling and advice centres.

Sexual harassment

The student should be advised to make a formal complaint in writing, which will be investigated by the Human Resources Department of the university. Student counselling is also available for support. GPs can approach the British Medical Association and defence organisations for confidential advice.

Crime

If a crime is discovered the police should be involved and the GMC notified. Students should be made aware of the seriousness of a criminal record; fare dodging, plagiarism and drug and alcohol-related offences may all result in a Fitness to Practise hearing at the university.

___ Conclusions

Mentoring requires empathy; for this to be sustained the mentor needs to be self-aware. Over-involvement with the mentee will cause personal distress and the mentor will not be in a good position to make objective decisions. Mentors, like other doctors, require support for themselves, which may be provided by their own mentor or in a group setting. Mentors may find it helpful to meet together to discuss difficult problems. Mentors do not work in isolation. They are part of a support network and they should be ready to involve others if they are struggling with a difficult issue.

Key points

Mentors need to keep to professional boundaries.

Confidentiality can create problems for the mentor.

There are situations where a rapid response is essential.

Mentors need to have access to support for themselves.

___ References

1 Long J. The Dark Side of Mentoring. AARE conference 1994. www.aare.edu.au/data/publications/1994/longj94030.pdf   [accessed 25 June 2014].

2 Kalen S, Panzer S, Silen C. The core of mentorship: medical students' experiences of one-to-one mentoring in a clinical environment. *Advances in Health Sciences Education* 2012; **17(3)**: 389–401.

3 General Medical Council. *Good Medical Practice.* London: GMC, 2013.

4 Centre for Suicide Research. *Assessment of Suicide Risk in People with Depression.* Oxford: University of Oxford, n.d., http://cebmh.warne.ox.ac.uk/csr/Clinical_guide_assessing_suicide_risk.pdf   [accessed 25 June 2014].

CONCLUDING REMARKS

Mentoring can help an individual to develop his or her professional practice both practically and emotionally. Practically, the individual may be better equipped to cope with competing demands and to prioritise more effectively. Emotionally he or she may have renewed enthusiasm for work and no longer feel stressed. Mentoring has been shown to reduce stress and help individuals adapt to change. Psychological benefits include improved job satisfaction, a better work–life balance and improved personal and professional relationships. Individuals will be better equipped to set personal objectives and take part in reflective learning. Reflection becomes a way of increasing self-awareness rather than a chore. Mentoring improves productivity, job satisfaction, career preparation and workplace learning.[1]

In a broader sense mentoring also helps recruitment, retention and improves the morale in the organisation. In one university studied over five years of student entry, among 1188 students who enrolled for medicine, 73 (6%) failed to qualify; 46 dropped out in the first two years, 17 in year 3 and ten in the final two years.[2] These figures represent a large financial cost and, more importantly, a psychological blow to the students and to their families. The NHS and patients benefit from the provision of mentoring because staff who are less stressed deliver better patient care. The scarcity of formal mentoring programmes in the NHS and universities is in striking contrast to the overwhelming evidence of its importance.[1] Mentoring needs to be recognised as a core teaching activity, not the hobby of a few enthusiasts. During their careers mentees may choose more than one mentor from different disciplines.

Mentors support their mentee through the transitions of their career. They help mentees to find their way through the hidden curriculum of the profession towards establishing their own individual professional identity.[3] The mentor recognises that these transitions are not simply a matter of accumulating more knowledge; the professional self and the personal self are intertwined. The help and encouragement the mentor offers the student or doctor must be of a quality high enough to support both professional and personal issues. Artificial divisions between academic and pastoral support should be rejected, as these 'divisions' are often created to make the task easier for a mentor rather than to address the real needs of the mentee.[3]

The mentor's role varies to meet the needs of each individual mentee in an evolving relationship. As this relationship deepens the mentee becomes more independent as he or she reaches his or her full potential. Mentoring should be valued by the organisation responsible for the training of doctors and students. Mentors need recognition, training, a forum to express their concerns and protected time for mentoring. Mentoring should not be relegated to a remedial service for struggling students or doctors in difficulty but should be part of every student's and doctor's training. If mentorship is only offered when there are performance problems it will be resisted. Awareness of the potential benefits of mentoring needs to be raised amongst doctors so that they know what can be gained from the relationship. It is hoped that this book will encourage doctors in a variety of settings to act as mentors for their colleagues.

Mentorship engenders professional development not only for the mentee but also for the mentor him or herself; it is fulfilling work that enhances self-awareness. Students and doctors in training can teach a mentor by showing how they cope with adversity, embrace change and regain an enthusiasm for their work. Mentoring may be a short relationship, during the undergraduate years, or may last for many years in a relationship of friendship and mutual respect. After working through a minefield of problems it is heartening that good mentors are remembered with gratitude, by so many students and doctors, for the time they spent listening.

_____ **References**

1   Driessen EW, Overeem K, van der Vleuten CPM. Get yourself a mentor. *Medical Education* 2011; **45(5)**: 438–9.

2   Yates J. When did they leave, and why? A retrospective case study of attrition at the Nottingham undergraduate medical course. *BMC Medical Education* 2012; **12**: 43.

3   Freeman R. Faculty mentoring programmes. *Medical Education* 2000; **34(7)**: 507–8.

__Index

Note: page numbers in *italics* refer to figures and tables.